FITNESS FUNDAMENTALS

A Beginner's Guide to Effective Exercise

SAMUEL JAMES

DEDICATION

To my family, whose unwavering support and love have been my foundation,

To my friends, who have inspired and encouraged me every step of the way,

And to all the dreamers and doers, who strive for success and never give up,

This book is dedicated to you.

May it be a guide and a source of inspiration on your journey to achieving your dreams.

With heartfelt gratitude.

TABLE OF CONTENT

INTRODUCTION

Overview of Fitness Fundamentals

Embarking on a fitness journey can be both exciting and daunting, especially for beginners. "Fitness Fundamentals: A Beginner's Guide to Effective Exercise" is designed to demystify the world of exercise and provide you with a solid foundation to build a lifelong fitness habit.

The Importance of Starting an Exercise Routine:

Starting an exercise routine is a pivotal step towards improving your overall health and well-being. Regular physical activity is crucial for maintaining physical and mental health. Here's why initiating an exercise regimen is essential:

1. **Health Benefits:**
   - **Cardiovascular Health:** Regular exercise strengthens the heart and improves blood circulation, reducing the risk of cardiovascular diseases such as heart attacks, strokes, and high blood pressure.
   - **Weight Management:** Physical activity helps control weight by burning calories and building muscle, which increases metabolism.

- **Bone and Muscle Strength:** Weight-bearing exercises strengthen bones and muscles, reducing the risk of osteoporosis and frailty as you age.
- **Mental Health:** Exercise has been proven to reduce symptoms of depression, anxiety, and stress. It promotes the release of endorphins, which are natural mood lifters.

2. **Lifestyle Benefits:**
   - **Increased Energy Levels:** Regular exercise boosts energy levels by improving muscle strength and endurance.
   - **Better Sleep:** Engaging in physical activities helps regulate sleep patterns, leading to deeper and more restful sleep.
   - **Improved Cognitive Function:** Exercise enhances brain function, improves memory, and increases the ability to focus and concentrate.
   - **Enhanced Self-Esteem:** Achieving fitness goals, however small, can boost your confidence and self-esteem.

3. **Disease Prevention:**
   - **Chronic Disease Management:** Exercise helps manage chronic conditions like diabetes, arthritis, and high cholesterol.
   - **Immune System Support:** Regular physical activity can strengthen the immune system, making you less susceptible to illnesses.

The Benefits of Regular Physical Activity:

Regular physical activity offers a myriad of benefits that extend beyond physical health. Here are some key advantages:

1. **Physical Health:**
   - **Improved Flexibility and Balance:** Regular exercise improves flexibility and balance, reducing the risk of falls and injuries.
   - **Enhanced Muscular Endurance:** Physical activities build and maintain muscle mass, essential for daily activities and overall strength.
   - **Healthy Body Composition:** Exercise helps maintain a healthy ratio of fat to muscle, contributing to a leaner and healthier body composition.
2. **Mental and Emotional Health:**
   - **Stress Relief:** Exercise acts as a natural stress reliever by reducing the levels of stress hormones and promoting relaxation.
   - **Enhanced Mood:** The release of endorphins during exercise can create feelings of happiness and euphoria.
   - **Social Interaction:** Participating in group activities or fitness classes can foster social connections and reduce feelings of loneliness.
3. **Longevity:**

- o **Increased Lifespan:** Studies have shown that regular physical activity can extend lifespan by reducing the risk of chronic diseases and promoting overall health.

The Purpose and Structure of the Book:

"Fitness Fundamentals: A Beginner's Guide to Effective Exercise" is meticulously designed to guide you through the process of establishing a consistent and effective exercise routine. The book is structured to provide you with comprehensive knowledge, practical tips, and motivational insights to help you succeed in your fitness journey. Here's what you can expect:

1. **Foundational Knowledge:**
   - o **Chapter 1: Getting Started:** This chapter will cover the basics of setting realistic fitness goals, understanding your fitness level, and the importance of a balanced diet.
   - o **Chapter 2: Understanding Exercise Types:** Learn about different types of exercises, including cardiovascular, strength training, flexibility, and balance exercises.
2. **Practical Guidance:**
   - o **Chapter 3: Creating Your Workout Plan:** Step-by-step instructions on how to create a personalized workout plan that suits your lifestyle and goals.

- o **Chapter 4: Equipment and Facilities:** Information on the essential equipment you might need and how to utilize fitness facilities effectively.
3. **Detailed Exercise Instructions:**
   - o **Chapter 5: Beginner Workouts:** Detailed descriptions and illustrations of beginner-friendly exercises for different parts of the body.
   - o **Chapter 6: Progressing Your Workouts:** How to gradually increase the intensity and complexity of your workouts as you become more fit.
4. **Safety and Recovery:**
   - o **Chapter 7: Avoiding Injuries:** Tips on how to exercise safely and prevent common injuries.
   - o **Chapter 8: The Importance of Recovery:** Understanding the role of rest and recovery in your fitness routine.
5. **Motivation and Mindset:**
   - o **Chapter 9: Staying Motivated:** Strategies for staying motivated and overcoming common obstacles.
   - o **Chapter 10: Building a Lifelong Fitness Habit:** Tips on how to make exercise a permanent part of your lifestyle.

Why Exercise Matters

Physical, Mental, and Emotional Benefits of Exercise

Exercise is a cornerstone of a healthy lifestyle, offering numerous benefits that extend beyond just physical health. Understanding these benefits can help motivate you to incorporate regular physical activity into your daily routine.

Physical Benefits:

1. **Improved Cardiovascular Health:**
   - **Heart Strength:** Regular exercise strengthens the heart, making it more efficient at pumping blood, which can reduce the risk of heart diseases, such as heart attacks and strokes.
   - **Blood Pressure:** Physical activity helps lower blood pressure by improving the heart's efficiency and reducing the stiffness of arteries.
   - **Cholesterol Levels:** Exercise can increase high-density lipoprotein (HDL) cholesterol, the "good" cholesterol, and decrease low-density lipoprotein (LDL) cholesterol, the "bad" cholesterol.
2. **Weight Management:**
   - **Calorie Burn:** Physical activity helps burn calories, contributing to weight loss or maintenance. Even low-intensity activities, like walking, can help in weight management.
   - **Metabolism Boost:** Exercise increases muscle mass, which in turn boosts metabolism, allowing you to burn more calories even at rest.

3. **Muscle and Bone Health:**
   - **Strength and Endurance:** Regular strength training exercises build muscle mass and improve endurance, making daily activities easier and reducing the risk of falls and injuries.
   - **Bone Density:** Weight-bearing exercises, such as walking and strength training, increase bone density and reduce the risk of osteoporosis.
4. **Improved Flexibility and Balance:**
   - **Range of Motion:** Stretching exercises improve flexibility, allowing for a greater range of motion and reducing the risk of injuries.
   - **Stability:** Balance exercises strengthen core muscles and improve stability, which is crucial for preventing falls, especially in older adults.

Mental Benefits:

1. **Enhanced Cognitive Function:**
   - **Brain Health:** Exercise increases blood flow to the brain, promoting the growth of new brain cells and enhancing brain function. It can improve memory, attention, and processing speed.
   - **Neuroplasticity:** Physical activity supports neuroplasticity, the brain's ability to adapt and form new neural connections, which is crucial for learning and cognitive resilience.

2. **Stress Reduction:**
   - **Endorphin Release:** Exercise triggers the release of endorphins, the body's natural mood elevators, which can reduce stress and create a sense of well-being.
   - **Relaxation:** Activities like yoga and tai chi incorporate mindfulness and deep breathing, helping to calm the mind and reduce stress levels.
3. **Improved Sleep:**
   - **Sleep Quality:** Regular exercise can help you fall asleep faster and deepen your sleep. It regulates your circadian rhythm, the body's internal clock, promoting better sleep patterns.
   - **Sleep Disorders:** Physical activity can alleviate symptoms of sleep disorders such as insomnia and sleep apnea.

Emotional Benefits:

1. **Mood Enhancement:**
   - **Depression and Anxiety:** Exercise has been shown to reduce symptoms of depression and anxiety. It provides a distraction from negative thoughts and promotes a sense of accomplishment.
   - **Self-Esteem:** Achieving fitness goals, no matter how small, can boost self-confidence and self-esteem.
2. **Social Interaction:**

- o **Community and Support:** Group activities and fitness classes offer opportunities to meet new people and build a supportive community, reducing feelings of loneliness and isolation.
- o **Motivation:** Social interactions during exercise can provide motivation and encouragement, making it more likely to stick to your fitness routine.

The Role of Exercise in Overall Health and Wellness

Exercise plays a critical role in maintaining and enhancing overall health and wellness. It is a key component of a holistic approach to health that includes a balanced diet, adequate sleep, and stress management.

Prevention of Chronic Diseases:

- **Diabetes:** Regular physical activity helps regulate blood sugar levels and improves insulin sensitivity, reducing the risk of type 2 diabetes.
- **Hypertension:** Exercise helps lower high blood pressure and reduces the risk of developing hypertension.
- **Cancer:** Physical activity has been linked to a lower risk of certain cancers, including breast, colon, and lung cancer.

Boosting the Immune System:

- **Immune Function:** Regular exercise can enhance the immune system, making it more effective at fighting off infections and illnesses.
- **Inflammation:** Exercise reduces chronic inflammation, which is linked to many diseases, including heart disease, diabetes, and cancer.

Longevity:

- **Life Expectancy:** Studies have shown that regular physical activity can extend life expectancy by reducing the risk of chronic diseases and improving overall health.

Quality of Life:

- **Daily Functioning:** Exercise improves physical function and mobility, making daily tasks easier and enhancing the quality of life.
- **Mental Well-being:** Regular physical activity promotes mental well-being, helping to maintain a positive outlook on life.

Addressing Common Misconceptions About Fitness

There are several misconceptions about fitness that can hinder people from starting or maintaining an exercise routine. Addressing these misconceptions can help you approach fitness with a more informed and positive mindset.

Misconception 1: "You Need to Exercise for Hours to See Benefits":

- **Reality:** Even short bursts of physical activity can be beneficial. The key is consistency. Incorporating just 30 minutes of moderate exercise most days of the week can significantly improve health.

Misconception 2: "Exercise is Only for Weight Loss":

- **Reality:** While exercise can aid in weight management, its benefits extend far beyond weight loss. It improves cardiovascular health, mental well-being, muscle and bone strength, and overall longevity.

Misconception 3: "You Have to Go to the Gym to Exercise":

- **Reality:** Exercise can be done anywhere. Activities like walking, jogging, home workouts, and recreational sports can be just as effective as gym workouts.

Misconception 4: "You Need to Be Young and Fit to Start Exercising":

- **Reality:** It's never too late to start exercising. Physical activity is beneficial at any age and fitness level. Starting slow and gradually increasing intensity is key to avoiding injury and building fitness.

Misconception 5: "Exercise is Only for Athletes":

- **Reality:** Exercise is for everyone. Regardless of your athletic ability, incorporating regular physical activity into your routine can enhance your health and well-being.

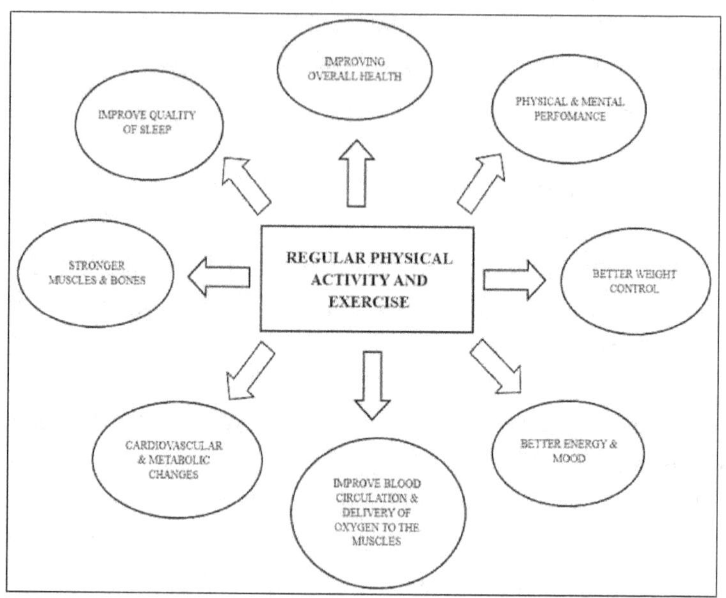

Part 1: Getting Started

Chapter 1: Setting Your Fitness Goals

Setting fitness goals is a crucial first step in any exercise journey. Goals give you direction, motivation, and a sense of purpose. They help you measure your progress and celebrate your achievements. This chapter will guide you through the process of setting effective fitness goals that are tailored to your needs and aspirations.

Understanding the Importance of Goal-Setting

1. Provides Direction and Focus:

- **Clear Path:** Having specific goals helps you create a structured plan. It provides a roadmap that outlines what you need to do to achieve your desired outcome.
- **Focus:** Goals help you concentrate on what's important. They prevent you from getting sidetracked by irrelevant activities or distractions.

2. Motivation and Commitment:

- **Increased Motivation:** Goals keep you motivated. They give you something to strive for and look forward to. The sense of accomplishment you feel when you achieve a goal can be a powerful motivator to keep going.

- **Commitment:** When you set goals, you make a commitment to yourself. This commitment can help you stay dedicated to your fitness routine, even when it gets tough.

3. Measure Progress:

- **Tracking Progress:** Goals provide benchmarks to measure your progress. They help you see how far you've come and what you need to do to reach your destination.
- **Adjustments:** By regularly reviewing your goals, you can identify areas where you need to make adjustments to your plan or effort.

4. Builds Self-Esteem and Confidence:

- **Achievement:** Every goal you achieve boosts your self-esteem and confidence. It proves to you that you are capable of setting and achieving objectives, which can be empowering.

How to Set SMART Goals

SMART goals are specific, measurable, achievable, relevant, and time-bound. This framework ensures that your goals are clear and attainable.

1. Specific:

- **Clear and Precise:** Your goals should be specific, clear, and well-defined. Avoid vague goals like "get fit." Instead, specify what you want to achieve, such as "run a 5K" or "lose 10 pounds."

- **Detailed Plan:** A specific goal outlines the steps you need to take to achieve it. For example, "I will run three times a week for 30 minutes each session to prepare for a 5K race."

2. Measurable:

- **Track Progress:** Your goals should be measurable so you can track your progress. Include specific criteria that will help you measure your success.
- **Quantifiable:** Use numbers and deadlines. For example, "I will increase my bench press by 10 pounds in three months."

3. Achievable:

- **Realistic:** Your goals should be challenging yet achievable. Setting unrealistic goals can lead to frustration and demotivation.
- **Attainable:** Consider your current fitness level, resources, and time. Ensure your goal is within reach with effort and commitment.

4. Relevant:

- **Aligned with Values:** Your goals should be relevant to your interests and aligned with your overall objectives. They should matter to you personally.
- **Purposeful:** Ask yourself why the goal is important and how it fits into your broader life

plans. For example, if you want to improve your health, a relevant goal might be "exercise for 30 minutes daily to reduce stress and improve cardiovascular health."

5. Time-Bound:

- **Deadline:** Set a deadline for your goals. This creates a sense of urgency and helps you stay focused.
- **Time Frame:** Specify a time frame for achieving your goal. For example, "I will lose 10 pounds in three months by following a balanced diet and exercising five times a week."

Examples of Short-Term and Long-Term Fitness Goals

1. Short-Term Goals:

- **Increase Workout Frequency:** "I will work out at the gym four times a week for the next month."
- **Improve Flexibility:** "I will practice yoga for 20 minutes every morning for the next two weeks."
- **Healthy Eating:** "I will drink eight glasses of water daily and reduce my sugar intake for the next 30 days."
- **Cardio Fitness:** "I will jog for 20 minutes three times a week for the next month."
- **Strength Training:** "I will add 10 pounds to my squat within six weeks."

2. Long-Term Goals:

- **Weight Loss:** "I will lose 30 pounds over the next year by following a balanced diet and exercising regularly."
- **Running a Marathon:** "I will train for and complete a marathon within the next 12 months."
- **Muscle Gain:** "I will gain 15 pounds of muscle mass over the next year by following a strength training program and eating a high-protein diet."
- **Consistent Routine:** "I will maintain a consistent exercise routine for at least one year, including a mix of cardio, strength training, and flexibility exercises."
- **Health Improvement:** "I will lower my blood pressure to a healthy range within six months by exercising regularly and improving my diet."

Putting It All Together

Setting fitness goals is an empowering process that helps you take control of your health and fitness journey. By understanding the importance of goal-setting and following the SMART framework, you can create clear, achievable, and motivating goals that will guide you toward a healthier and more active lifestyle. As you progress, remember to celebrate your achievements, no matter how small, and adjust your goals as needed to continue challenging yourself and maintaining your commitment to fitness.

Chapter 2: Understanding Basic Exercise Principles

Embarking on a fitness journey involves more than just moving your body; it requires an understanding of foundational exercise principles to maximize your results and minimize the risk of injury. This chapter delves into three critical exercise principles: overload, progression, and specificity. It also highlights the essential roles of consistency and recovery in achieving fitness goals and emphasizes the importance of proper warm-up and cool-down routines.

The Principles of Overload, Progression, and Specificity

1. Overload

Definition: Overload refers to the need to increase the demand on your body to make it adapt and become stronger. Without progressively challenging your body, your fitness levels will plateau.

Application:

- **Increasing Intensity:** Gradually increase the intensity of your workouts by adding more weight, increasing resistance, or upping the speed of your exercises.
- **Increasing Duration:** Extend the length of your workout sessions or the time spent on each exercise.

- **Increasing Frequency:** Add more workout sessions to your weekly routine.

Benefits:

- **Muscle Growth:** Overloading muscles by lifting heavier weights leads to hypertrophy (muscle growth).
- **Improved Endurance:** Longer cardio sessions improve cardiovascular endurance.
- **Increased Strength:** Higher resistance challenges muscle strength.

2. Progression

Definition: Progression involves gradually increasing the intensity, duration, or frequency of exercise over time. This ensures continuous improvement and adaptation by the body.

Application:

- **Structured Plan:** Create a workout plan that gradually increases the workload over weeks and months.
- **Regular Assessment:** Periodically assess your performance and adjust your plan to ensure continued progress.
- **Incremental Increases:** Make small, manageable increases in weight, reps, sets, or duration to avoid injury and ensure steady progress.

Benefits:

- **Sustainable Growth:** Ensures steady, sustainable improvement without overwhelming the body.
- **Prevents Plateaus:** Keeps the body continuously adapting and improving, preventing fitness plateaus.
- **Enhanced Motivation:** Visible progress keeps you motivated and committed to your fitness goals.

3. Specificity

Definition: Specificity means that the type of exercise you do should be relevant and appropriate to your fitness goals. Your body adapts specifically to the type of exercise you perform.

Application:

- **Goal-Oriented Workouts:** Tailor your workouts to match your specific fitness goals. For example, if you want to build muscle, focus on strength training; if you aim to run a marathon, prioritize endurance training.
- **Sport-Specific Training:** Athletes should train in ways that mimic the movements and demands of their sport.
- **Targeted Exercises:** Choose exercises that target the muscle groups and energy systems required for your goals.

Benefits:

- **Optimal Results:** Achieve the best results by focusing on exercises that directly support your goals.
- **Efficient Training:** Maximize your workout efficiency by prioritizing relevant exercises.
- **Improved Performance:** Enhance performance in specific activities or sports by training in a specific manner.

The Role of Consistency and Recovery in Fitness

1. Consistency

Definition: Consistency involves maintaining a regular exercise routine over time. Sporadic or infrequent workouts are less effective and can lead to setbacks.

Application:

- **Regular Schedule:** Establish a consistent workout schedule that fits your lifestyle and stick to it.
- **Long-Term Commitment:** View fitness as a long-term commitment rather than a short-term goal.
- **Habit Formation:** Build exercise into your daily or weekly routine until it becomes a habit.

Benefits:

- **Steady Progress:** Regular exercise leads to gradual and sustained improvements in fitness.

- **Enhanced Discipline:** Consistency builds discipline, making it easier to stay committed to your fitness routine.
- **Preventing Setbacks:** Regular activity reduces the likelihood of losing progress and having to start over.

2. Recovery

Definition: Recovery is the period needed for the body to repair and strengthen itself between workouts. It is during this time that muscles rebuild and grow stronger.

Application:

- **Rest Days:** Incorporate rest days into your workout schedule to allow your body to recover.
- **Active Recovery:** Engage in low-intensity activities like walking, stretching, or yoga to promote blood flow and aid recovery.
- **Proper Sleep and Nutrition:** Ensure adequate sleep and nutrition to support recovery and muscle repair.

Benefits:

- **Injury Prevention:** Adequate recovery prevents overuse injuries and reduces the risk of burnout.
- **Improved Performance:** Well-rested muscles perform better, leading to more effective workouts.

- **Enhanced Adaptation:** Recovery allows your body to adapt to the stress of exercise, leading to greater strength and endurance.

The Importance of Warm-Up and Cool-Down Routines

1. Warm-Up

Definition: A warm-up is a set of exercises performed before the main workout to prepare your body for physical activity. It gradually increases your heart rate, blood flow to muscles, and joint mobility.

Application:

- **Dynamic Stretching:** Perform dynamic stretches that mimic the movements of your workout to warm up the muscles and joints.
- **Gradual Intensity:** Start with low-intensity exercises and gradually increase the intensity to prepare your body for the workout.
- **Specific Movements:** Focus on warming up the muscle groups that will be used during the main workout.

Benefits:

- **Injury Prevention:** Warm muscles and joints are less prone to injury.
- **Improved Performance:** A proper warm-up enhances muscle performance and coordination.
- **Increased Flexibility:** Dynamic stretching increases the range of motion and flexibility.

2. Cool-Down

Definition: A cool-down is a set of exercises performed after the main workout to gradually reduce heart rate and relax the muscles. It aids in the recovery process.

Application:

- **Static Stretching:** Perform static stretches to lengthen and relax the muscles.
- **Gradual Decrease:** Slowly decrease the intensity of your activity to allow your heart rate to return to normal.
- **Deep Breathing:** Incorporate deep breathing exercises to relax and calm the body.

Benefits:

- **Reduced Soreness:** A proper cool-down helps reduce muscle soreness and stiffness.
- **Enhanced Recovery:** Gradual reduction in activity aids in the removal of metabolic waste and promotes faster recovery.
- **Flexibility Improvement:** Static stretching post-workout can improve overall flexibility.

Chapter 3: Building a Fitness Routine

Creating a fitness routine that is balanced, comprehensive, and tailored to your individual needs is crucial for achieving your health and wellness goals. This chapter will guide you through the process of developing an effective exercise program, understanding the different types of exercise, and implementing sample weekly workout plans designed specifically for beginners.

How to Create a Balanced Exercise Program

A well-rounded fitness routine should incorporate various types of exercise to ensure all aspects of physical fitness are addressed. Here's how to create a balanced exercise program:

1. Assess Your Current Fitness Level

Before you begin, evaluate your current fitness level to establish a baseline. This can involve:

- **Self-Assessment:** Reflect on your current physical activity, any limitations, and overall health.
- **Fitness Tests:** Consider simple fitness tests like measuring your resting heart rate, testing your flexibility with a sit-and-reach test, or doing a timed walk/run to gauge cardiovascular endurance.

2. Set Clear Fitness Goals

Establishing clear and achievable fitness goals is essential. Use the SMART criteria to ensure your goals are:

- **Specific:** Clearly define what you want to achieve.
- **Measurable:** Ensure your progress can be tracked.
- **Achievable:** Set realistic goals within your current capabilities.
- **Relevant:** Align your goals with your overall fitness aspirations.
- **Time-bound:** Set a timeframe to achieve your goals.

3. Plan for All Components of Fitness

A balanced exercise program should include:

- **Cardiovascular Exercise:** Activities that increase your heart rate and improve heart and lung health.
- **Strength Training:** Exercises that build and tone muscles.
- **Flexibility Exercises:** Stretching routines that improve the range of motion of your muscles and joints.
- **Balance Exercises:** Activities that enhance stability and coordination.

4. Create a Weekly Schedule

Plan your workouts for the week, ensuring you have a mix of different types of exercise. Aim to balance intensity and rest, and schedule workouts at times that suit your lifestyle to ensure consistency.

5. Monitor Progress and Adjust

Regularly review your progress and make adjustments as needed. Track your workouts, note improvements, and adapt your routine to continue challenging your body and avoiding plateaus.

The Different Types of Exercise

Understanding the different types of exercise is essential to creating a comprehensive fitness program. Each type plays a unique role in improving your overall health and fitness:

1. Cardiovascular Exercise

Definition: Cardiovascular (cardio) exercise involves activities that increase your heart rate and breathing. It is essential for improving heart and lung function, burning calories, and enhancing overall endurance.

Examples:

- Running or jogging
- Cycling
- Swimming
- Brisk walking
- Dancing
- Jump rope

Benefits:

- Improves cardiovascular health
- Aids in weight management
- Enhances lung capacity and stamina
- Reduces the risk of chronic diseases

2. Strength Training

Definition: Strength training involves exercises that build muscle strength and endurance. This type of exercise is critical for maintaining muscle mass, enhancing metabolism, and improving bone density.

Examples:

- Weight lifting
- Bodyweight exercises (push-ups, squats, lunges)
- Resistance band exercises
- Pilates
- Using weight machines

Benefits:

- Increases muscle strength and tone
- Boosts metabolism
- Improves bone health
- Enhances functional fitness for daily activities

3. Flexibility Exercises

Definition: Flexibility exercises involve stretching activities that improve the range of motion of your muscles and joints. Flexibility is important for overall mobility and reducing the risk of injuries.

Examples:

- Static stretching
- Dynamic stretching
- Yoga
- Tai Chi

Benefits:

- Enhances flexibility and range of motion
- Reduces muscle stiffness and soreness
- Decreases the risk of injuries
- Improves posture and alignment

4. Balance Exercises

Definition: Balance exercises are designed to improve stability and coordination. These exercises are particularly important for older adults to prevent falls and maintain independence.

Examples:

- Standing on one leg
- Heel-to-toe walk
- Balance exercises on a stability ball
- Yoga
- Tai Chi

Benefits:

- Improves balance and coordination
- Enhances stability and reduces the risk of falls
- Strengthens core muscles

- Increases body awareness

Sample Weekly Workout Plans for Beginners

To help you get started, here are two sample weekly workout plans designed for beginners. These plans incorporate all types of exercise to ensure a balanced routine:

Sample Plan 1: Basic Starter Routine

Monday:

- **Cardio:** 30-minute brisk walk or light jog
- **Flexibility:** 10 minutes of static stretching

Tuesday:

- **Strength Training:** 20 minutes of bodyweight exercises (squats, push-ups, lunges)
- **Balance:** 10 minutes of balance exercises (standing on one leg, heel-to-toe walk)

Wednesday:

- **Rest Day:** Light activity like walking or gentle yoga

Thursday:

- **Cardio:** 30-minute cycling or swimming
- **Flexibility:** 10 minutes of dynamic stretching

Friday:

- **Strength Training:** 20 minutes of resistance band exercises
- **Balance:** 10 minutes of balance exercises (stability ball exercises, yoga poses)

Saturday:

- **Cardio:** 30-minute brisk walk or light jog
- **Flexibility:** 10 minutes of static stretching

Sunday:

- **Rest Day:** Light activity like walking or gentle yoga

Sample Plan 2: Progressive Routine

Monday:

- **Cardio:** 20-minute walk/jog intervals
- **Flexibility:** 10 minutes of yoga stretches

Tuesday:

- **Strength Training:** 25 minutes of weight lifting (light weights)
- **Balance:** 10 minutes of balance exercises (Tai Chi, stability ball exercises)

Wednesday:

- **Cardio:** 30-minute cycling
- **Flexibility:** 10 minutes of dynamic stretching

Thursday:

- **Strength Training:** 25 minutes of bodyweight exercises (planks, lunges, push-ups)
- **Balance:** 10 minutes of yoga poses for balance

Friday:

- **Cardio:** 30-minute brisk walk or swimming
- **Flexibility:** 10 minutes of static stretching

Saturday:

- **Strength Training:** 25 minutes of resistance band exercises
- **Balance:** 10 minutes of standing on one leg, heel-to-toe walk

Sunday:

- **Rest Day:** Gentle yoga or rest

Conclusion

Building a fitness routine involves understanding and incorporating various types of exercise into a balanced program that suits your lifestyle and goals. By setting clear goals, planning a diverse and consistent schedule, and regularly reviewing your progress, you can create a sustainable and effective fitness routine. Use the sample workout plans as a starting point, and feel free to adjust them based on your needs and preferences. With dedication and consistency, you'll reap the numerous benefits of a well-rounded fitness program.

Part 2: Types of Exercise

Chapter 4: Cardiovascular Exercise

Cardiovascular exercise, often referred to as "cardio," is a cornerstone of any effective fitness regimen. This chapter delves into the myriad benefits of cardiovascular fitness, explores various forms of cardio exercises, and provides practical guidance on how to start and progress in a cardio routine.

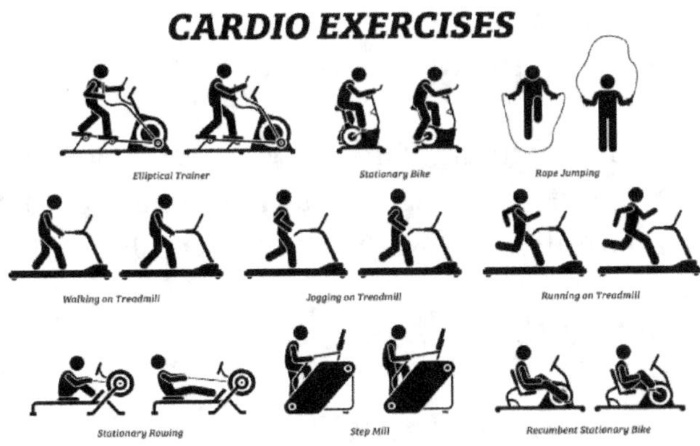

The Benefits of Cardiovascular Fitness

Cardiovascular fitness is crucial for maintaining overall health and well-being. Here are some of the key benefits:

1. Improved Heart Health

Cardio exercises strengthen the heart muscle, enabling it to pump blood more efficiently. This reduces the risk of heart disease, lowers blood pressure, and improves cholesterol levels.

2. Enhanced Lung Capacity

Regular cardio workouts improve lung capacity and efficiency, making it easier to breathe and increasing oxygen supply to the muscles.

3. Weight Management

Cardio exercises burn calories, helping you to maintain or lose weight. When combined with a balanced diet, cardio is an effective tool for weight management.

4. Increased Endurance and Stamina

Engaging in regular cardio workouts boosts your endurance and stamina, enabling you to perform everyday activities with greater ease and less fatigue.

5. Mental Health Benefits

Cardio exercise releases endorphins, often referred to as "feel-good" hormones. This can reduce stress, anxiety, and depression, leading to improved mental health and mood.

Different Forms of Cardio

There are various forms of cardiovascular exercise to suit different preferences and fitness levels. Here are some popular options:

1. Running

Benefits: Running is a high-impact exercise that strengthens the heart, burns calories, and tones muscles. **How to Start:** Begin with short distances and a combination of walking and running. Gradually increase your running time as your endurance improves. **Tips:** Invest in good running shoes, run on soft surfaces to reduce impact, and practice proper running form to avoid injuries.

2. Walking

Benefits: Walking is a low-impact exercise that is accessible to most people. It improves cardiovascular health, strengthens bones, and aids in weight management. **How to Start:** Start with short, brisk walks and gradually increase the duration and intensity. **Tips:** Maintain a good walking posture, use comfortable shoes, and try different terrains to keep it interesting.

3. Cycling

Benefits: Cycling is a low-impact exercise that improves cardiovascular fitness, strengthens leg muscles, and is easy on the joints. **How to Start:** Begin with short rides on flat terrain. Gradually increase the distance and incorporate hills as your fitness level improves. **Tips:** Ensure your bike is properly fitted, wear a helmet, and practice safe cycling habits.

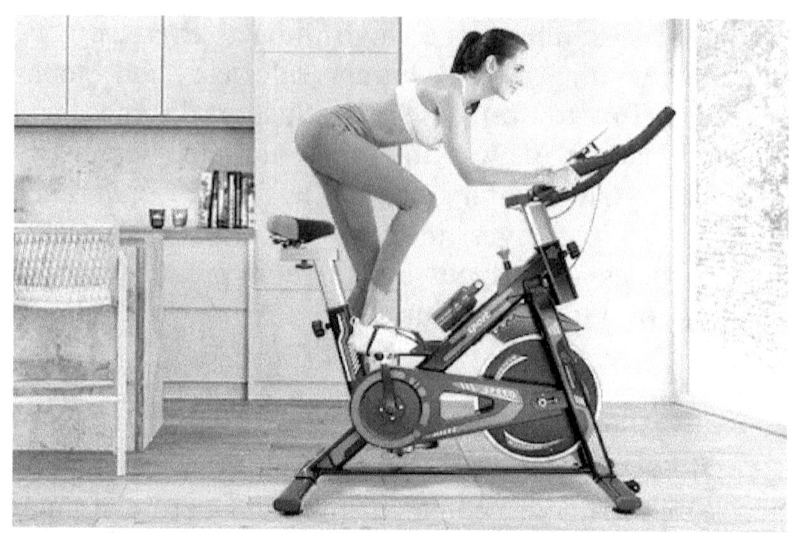

4. Swimming

Benefits: Swimming is a full-body workout that improves cardiovascular health, builds muscle strength, and is gentle on the joints. **How to Start:** Start with short swimming sessions, focusing on different strokes to work various muscle groups. **Tips:** Use proper technique to prevent injuries, and consider joining a swimming class for guidance.

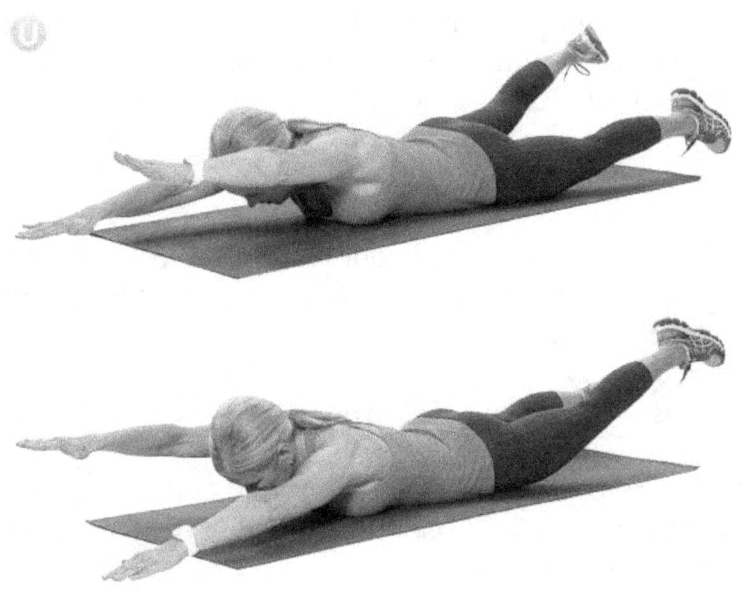

5. Group Classes

Benefits: Group classes, such as aerobics, Zumba, and spin classes, offer a structured and social way to improve cardiovascular fitness. **How to Start:** Choose a class that matches your fitness level and interests. Most gyms offer a variety of options. **Tips:** Attend regularly to build a routine, and don't be afraid to modify movements if needed.

How to Start and Progress in a Cardio Routine

Starting a cardio routine can be daunting, but with the right approach, it can be enjoyable and rewarding. Here's how to get started and progress:

1. Assess Your Fitness Level

Evaluate your current fitness level to choose an appropriate starting point. This can involve self-assessment or professional guidance.

2. Set Realistic Goals

Set SMART goals to give your cardio routine direction and purpose. For example, aim to walk briskly for 30 minutes five days a week.

3. Choose Activities You Enjoy

Select cardio exercises that you find enjoyable and sustainable. This increases the likelihood of sticking with your routine.

4. Start Slowly

Begin with low to moderate intensity workouts. Gradually increase the duration and intensity as your fitness improves.

5. Incorporate Variety

Mix different types of cardio to keep your workouts interesting and target different muscle groups. This also helps prevent overuse injuries.

6. Monitor Your Progress

Keep track of your workouts, noting the duration, intensity, and how you feel. This helps you see improvements and stay motivated.

7. Stay Consistent

Consistency is key to reaping the benefits of cardio exercise. Aim for at least 150 minutes of moderate-intensity cardio per week, as recommended by health guidelines.

8. Listen to Your Body

Pay attention to how your body responds to exercise. Rest when needed and avoid pushing yourself too hard, especially in the beginning.

Chapter 5: Strength Training

Strength training, also known as resistance training, is a crucial aspect of any well-rounded fitness routine. This chapter explores the importance of building muscle and strength, introduces basic strength training exercises, and provides detailed guidance on how to use various equipment, including free weights, resistance bands, and bodyweight exercises.

The Importance of Building Muscle and Strength

Strength training offers a multitude of benefits that extend beyond just building muscle. Here are some key reasons why incorporating strength training into your fitness regimen is essential:

1. Increased Muscle Mass

Strength training helps build and maintain muscle mass, which naturally declines with age. Increased muscle mass enhances physical appearance and overall strength.

2. Enhanced Metabolic Rate

Muscle tissue burns more calories at rest compared to fat tissue. Building muscle boosts your metabolic rate, aiding in weight management and fat loss.

3. Improved Bone Health

Resistance training increases bone density, reducing the risk of osteoporosis and fractures. This is particularly important as we age.

4. Enhanced Functional Strength

Building strength improves your ability to perform daily activities with ease, such as lifting groceries, climbing stairs, and carrying children.

5. Injury Prevention

Strengthening muscles, tendons, and ligaments enhances joint stability, reducing the likelihood of injuries.

6. Better Balance and Coordination

Strength training improves balance and coordination, which can help prevent falls and improve athletic performance.

7. Mental Health Benefits

Engaging in regular strength training can reduce symptoms of depression and anxiety, boost mood, and enhance overall mental well-being.

Basic Strength Training Exercises

To start building muscle and strength, it's essential to incorporate basic strength training exercises that target major muscle groups. Here are some foundational exercises:

1. Squats

Benefits: Squats target the quadriceps, hamstrings, glutes, and core, making them a comprehensive lower body exercise. **How to Perform:**

- Stand with your feet shoulder-width apart.
- Lower your body by bending your knees and hips, keeping your chest up and back straight.
- Go as low as you can while maintaining good form, then return to the starting position.

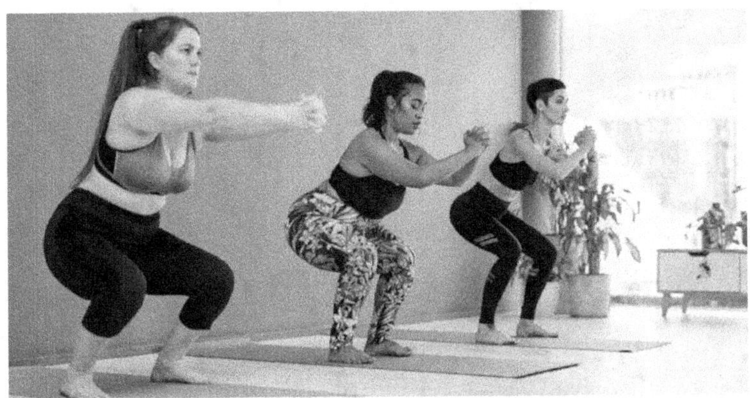

2. Lunges

Benefits: Lunges work the quadriceps, hamstrings, glutes, and calves while improving balance and coordination. **How to Perform:**

- Stand with your feet together.
- Step forward with one leg, lowering your hips until both knees are bent at about 90 degrees.
- Push back up to the starting position and repeat with the other leg.

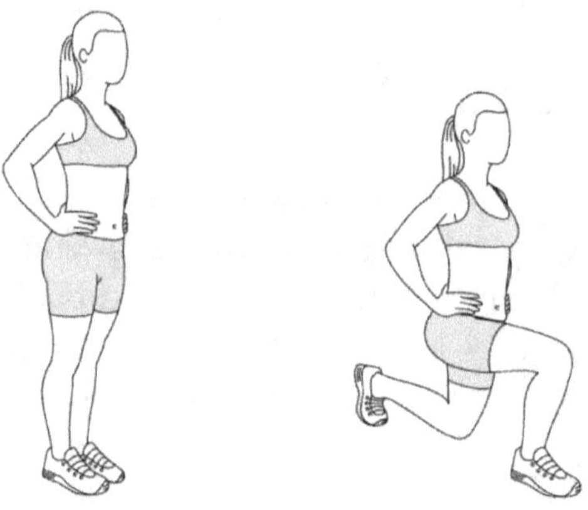

3. Push-Ups

Benefits: Push-ups strengthen the chest, shoulders, triceps, and core. **How to Perform:**

- Start in a plank position with your hands slightly wider than shoulder-width apart.

- Lower your body until your chest nearly touches the floor.
- Push back up to the starting position, keeping your body straight throughout the movement.

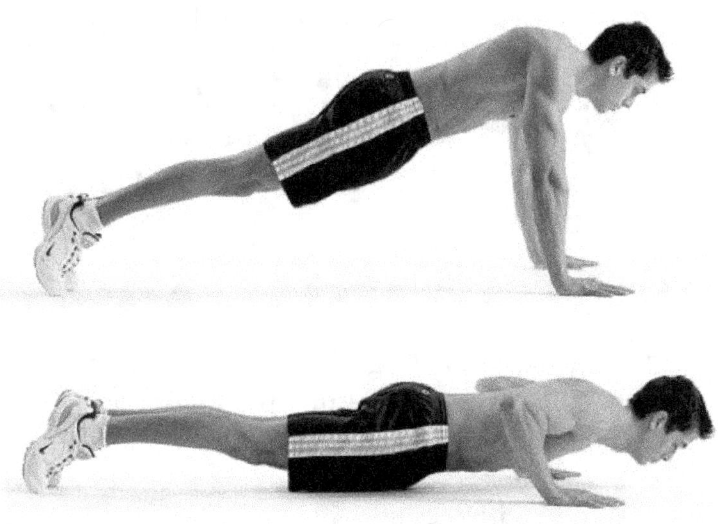

4. Planks

Benefits: Planks engage the core, shoulders, and back muscles, enhancing overall stability. **How to Perform:**

- Start in a push-up position, but with your weight on your forearms instead of your hands.
- Keep your body in a straight line from head to heels.
- Hold the position for as long as possible while maintaining good form.

The plank

- Elbows beneath shoulders
- Straight back
- Hold for two minutes

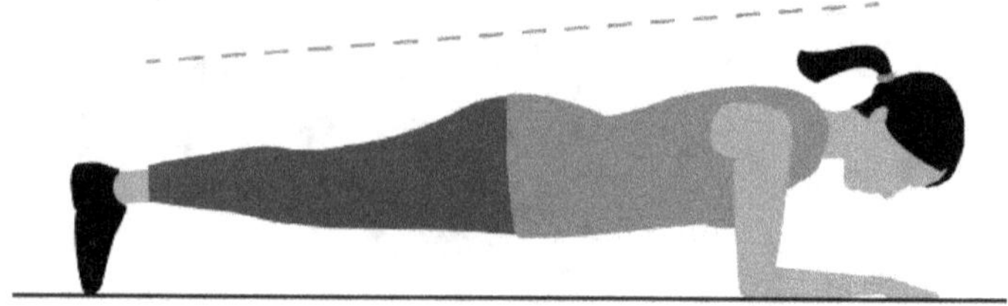

5. Deadlifts

Benefits: Deadlifts target the lower back, glutes, hamstrings, and core, making them a powerful full-body exercise. **How to Perform:**

- Stand with your feet hip-width apart and a barbell or dumbbells in front of you.
- Bend at the hips and knees to lower your body and grab the weight.
- Lift the weight by straightening your hips and knees, keeping your back straight throughout the movement.

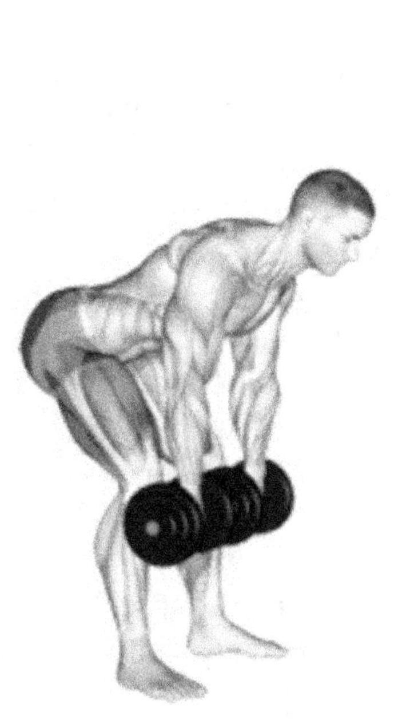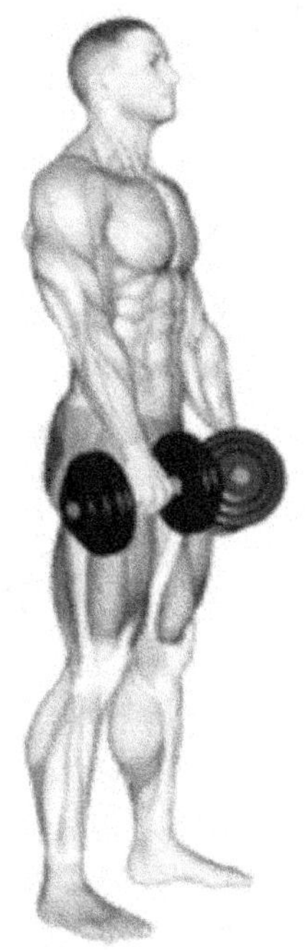

How to Use Free Weights, Resistance Bands, and Bodyweight Exercises

Incorporating different types of equipment can add variety to your strength training routine and target muscles in unique ways. Here's how to use free weights, resistance bands, and bodyweight exercises effectively:

1. Free Weights

Free weights, such as dumbbells and barbells, are versatile and effective for building strength. They require stabilizing muscles to engage, promoting overall muscle growth and balance.

Tips for Using Free Weights:

- **Start with Light Weights:** Begin with a weight that you can lift for 10-12 repetitions with proper form.
- **Progress Gradually:** Gradually increase the weight as you become stronger.
- **Focus on Form:** Proper form is crucial to prevent injuries and ensure effective muscle engagement. Consider seeking guidance from a trainer if you're new to weightlifting.

2. Resistance Bands

Resistance bands are portable, affordable, and versatile. They provide varying levels of resistance and can be used to target different muscle groups.

Tips for Using Resistance Bands:

- **Choose the Right Resistance:** Select a band that provides enough resistance to challenge you while allowing you to perform exercises with proper form.
- **Anchor Securely:** Ensure the band is securely anchored to avoid slipping or snapping.
- **Incorporate Variety:** Use bands for a range of exercises, such as bicep curls, shoulder presses, and leg lifts.

3. Bodyweight Exercises

Bodyweight exercises use your body as resistance and can be done anywhere without the need for equipment.

They are effective for building strength and improving functional fitness.

Tips for Bodyweight Exercises:

- **Master Basic Movements:** Focus on mastering basic movements like squats, push-ups, and planks before progressing to more advanced variations.
- **Increase Intensity:** Increase intensity by adding more repetitions, incorporating plyometric movements, or trying advanced variations (e.g., single-leg squats, decline push-ups).
- **Maintain Consistency:** Incorporate bodyweight exercises into your routine regularly to build and maintain strength.

Chapter 6: Flexibility and Mobility

Flexibility and mobility are essential components of a well-rounded fitness routine. While strength training and cardiovascular exercises often take center stage, flexibility and mobility play crucial roles in enhancing overall health, preventing injuries, and improving performance. This chapter explores the benefits of flexibility and mobility, introduces basic stretching exercises and techniques, and provides guidance on incorporating yoga and Pilates into your fitness routine.

The Benefits of Flexibility and Mobility for Overall Health

1. Improved Range of Motion

Flexibility and mobility exercises help increase the range of motion in your joints and muscles, allowing you to move more freely and comfortably. This improved range of motion can enhance performance in other forms of exercise and daily activities.

2. Reduced Risk of Injury

By increasing the elasticity of muscles and tendons, flexibility and mobility exercises can help prevent injuries. Flexible muscles are less likely to be strained or pulled, reducing the risk of exercise-related injuries.

3. Enhanced Muscle Coordination

Regular stretching and mobility work improve neuromuscular coordination, allowing your muscles to work more efficiently together. This can enhance your balance, stability, and overall movement quality.

4. Decreased Muscle Soreness and Tension

Stretching helps alleviate muscle soreness and tension by promoting blood flow to the muscles and facilitating the removal of metabolic waste products. This can lead to faster recovery after workouts.

5. Better Posture

Flexibility exercises, particularly those targeting the chest, shoulders, and hip flexors, can help correct muscle imbalances and improve posture. Better posture reduces strain on the spine and can alleviate back pain.

6. Enhanced Relaxation and Stress Relief

Stretching and mobility exercises can promote relaxation by reducing muscle tension and encouraging mindfulness. Activities like yoga incorporate breathing techniques that can lower stress levels and promote mental well-being.

Basic Stretching Exercises and Techniques

To reap the benefits of flexibility and mobility, it is essential to incorporate regular stretching exercises into your routine. Here are some basic stretching exercises and techniques to get you started:

1. Dynamic Stretching

Dynamic stretching involves moving parts of your body through a full range of motion in a controlled manner. These stretches are typically performed before a workout to prepare the muscles and joints for activity.

Examples of Dynamic Stretches:

- **Leg Swings:** Stand on one leg and swing the other leg forward and backward, gradually increasing the range of motion.
- **Arm Circles:** Extend your arms to the sides and make small, controlled circles, gradually increasing the size of the circles.

2. Static Stretching

Static stretching involves holding a stretch for a prolonged period, typically 15-60 seconds. These stretches are usually performed after a workout to help cool down and improve flexibility.

Examples of Static Stretches:

- **Hamstring Stretch:** Sit on the floor with one leg extended and the other bent. Reach towards your toes on the extended leg, holding the stretch.
- **Shoulder Stretch:** Bring one arm across your chest and use the opposite hand to gently pull the arm closer to your chest.

3. PNF Stretching

Proprioceptive Neuromuscular Facilitation (PNF) stretching involves a combination of stretching and contracting the muscle. This technique can improve flexibility more effectively than static stretching alone.

Example of PNF Stretching:

- **Hamstring PNF Stretch:** Lie on your back with one leg extended. Lift the other leg and hold it with your hands. Contract the hamstring by pushing against your hands for a few seconds, then relax and stretch further.

Incorporating Yoga and Pilates into Your Routine

Yoga and Pilates are excellent practices for improving flexibility and mobility while also offering additional benefits for overall health and fitness. Here's how you can incorporate them into your routine:

1. Yoga

Yoga combines physical postures, breathing exercises, and meditation to promote flexibility, strength, and relaxation. It is highly adaptable and can be modified to suit all fitness levels.

Benefits of Yoga:

- **Flexibility and Strength:** Yoga poses (asanas) stretch and strengthen muscles, enhancing overall flexibility and muscular endurance.
- **Stress Reduction:** The mindfulness and breathing techniques in yoga help reduce stress and promote relaxation.
- **Improved Balance:** Yoga poses often require balance and coordination, improving stability and proprioception.

Popular Yoga Poses for Flexibility:

- **Downward-Facing Dog (Adho Mukha Svanasana):** Stretches the hamstrings, calves, and shoulders.

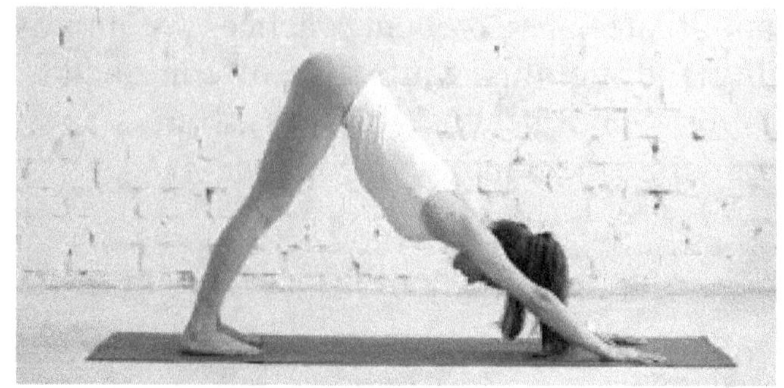

- **Seated Forward Bend (Paschimottanasana):** Stretches the hamstrings and lower back.

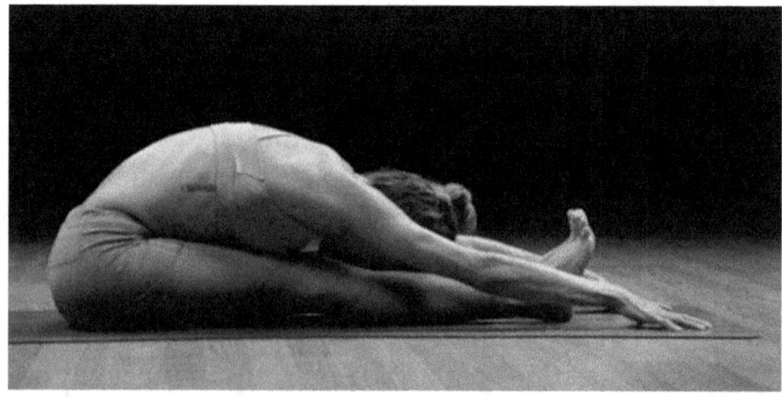

- **Cobra Pose (Bhujangasana):** Stretches the chest and abdominal muscles.

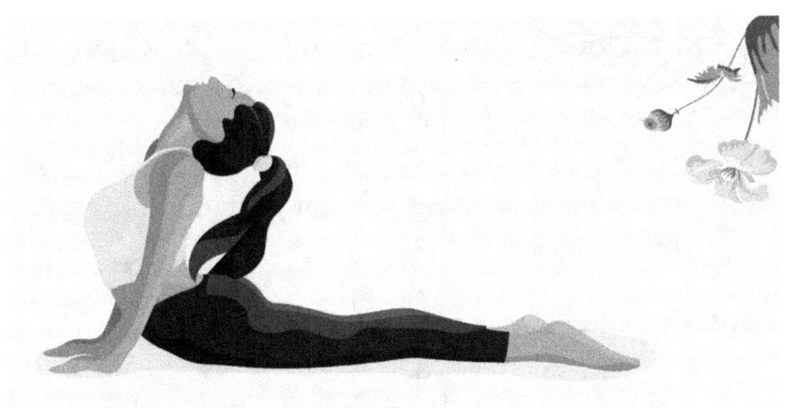

How to Get Started:

- **Find a Class:** Look for beginner yoga classes at local studios or online platforms.
- **Practice Regularly:** Aim to practice yoga at least 2-3 times per week to see improvements in flexibility and mobility.
- **Listen to Your Body:** Modify poses as needed and avoid pushing yourself into discomfort.

2. Pilates

Pilates focuses on core strength, flexibility, and overall body awareness. It involves controlled movements and emphasizes proper alignment and breathing.

Benefits of Pilates:

- **Core Strength:** Pilates exercises strengthen the deep core muscles, supporting better posture and stability.

- **Flexibility and Mobility:** The controlled, flowing movements in Pilates enhance flexibility and joint mobility.
- **Body Awareness:** Pilates improves body awareness, helping you understand and correct movement patterns.

Popular Pilates Exercises for Flexibility:

- **Roll-Up:** A core exercise that stretches the spine and hamstrings.
- **Spine Stretch Forward:** Stretches the back and hamstrings while promoting spinal mobility.
- **Leg Circles:** Improve hip flexibility and strengthen the core.

How to Get Started:

- **Join a Class:** Find a beginner Pilates class at a local studio or online.
- **Use Equipment:** Consider using a Pilates mat, resistance bands, or a Pilates reformer for added variety.
- **Focus on Form:** Pay attention to form and alignment to maximize the benefits and reduce the risk of injury.

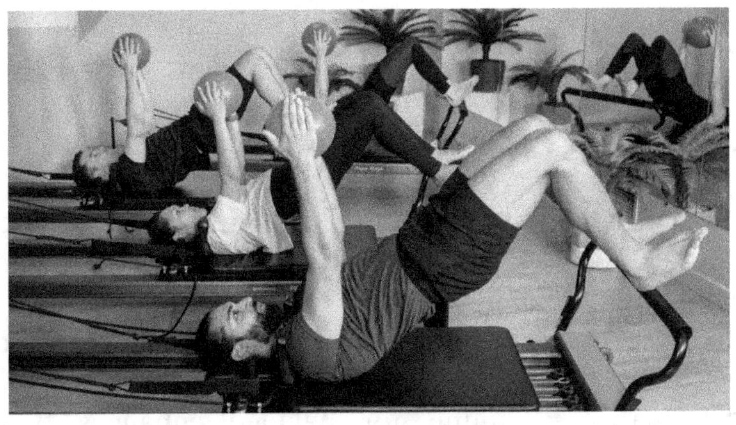

Chapter 7: Balance and Stability

Balance and stability are foundational components of overall fitness, playing crucial roles in daily activities and physical performance. They are often overlooked in exercise routines but are vital for maintaining a well-rounded fitness regimen. This chapter delves into the importance of balance and stability exercises, introduces simple exercises to improve balance and prevent falls, and provides guidance on integrating balance training into your workouts.

The Importance of Balance and Stability Exercises

1. Preventing Falls and Injuries

Balance and stability exercises are essential for preventing falls, especially in older adults. As we age, our balance naturally declines, increasing the risk of falls and related injuries. Regular balance training strengthens the muscles and improves the coordination needed to maintain stability, thereby reducing the risk of falls.

2. Enhancing Athletic Performance

Athletes benefit significantly from improved balance and stability. Whether it's a football player maintaining balance while dodging opponents, a dancer executing precise movements, or a runner stabilizing their stride, balance is critical for optimal performance. Training for balance enhances body control and coordination, which translates to better performance in sports and physical activities.

3. Improving Posture and Functional Movement

Good balance and stability contribute to better posture and functional movement. Proper balance training helps correct muscle imbalances, aligns the body correctly, and ensures that movements are efficient and safe. This is crucial for daily activities such as walking, climbing stairs, and lifting objects, making them easier and reducing the risk of injury.

4. Core Strength and Stability

Balance exercises often engage the core muscles, which are vital for maintaining stability. A strong core supports the spine, improves posture, and helps distribute weight evenly across the body. This not only enhances balance but also reduces the risk of back pain and other musculoskeletal issues.

Simple Exercises to Improve Balance and Prevent Falls

Incorporating simple balance exercises into your routine can have significant benefits. Here are some effective exercises to get you started:

1. Single-Leg Stand

This exercise is a basic but effective way to improve balance.

How to Perform:

- Stand with your feet hip-width apart.
- Shift your weight onto one foot and lift the other foot off the ground.
- Hold this position for as long as you can, aiming for 30 seconds to 1 minute.
- Switch legs and repeat.
- To increase the difficulty, try closing your eyes or standing on an unstable surface like a foam pad.

2. Heel-to-Toe Walk

The heel-to-toe walk is a simple exercise that improves balance and coordination.

How to Perform:

- Stand with your feet together.
- Step forward, placing the heel of one foot directly in front of the toes of the other foot.

- Continue walking in a straight line, placing each foot heel-to-toe.
- Focus on maintaining your balance and keeping your posture upright.
- Walk for 20 steps, turn around, and walk back.

3. Balance Board or Bosu Ball Exercises

Using a balance board or Bosu ball adds an element of instability, which challenges your balance and strengthens stabilizing muscles.

How to Perform:

- Stand on the balance board or Bosu ball with both feet.
- Shift your weight from side to side and front to back to maintain balance.
- As you become more comfortable, try performing exercises like squats or single-leg stands on the board or ball.

4. Tai Chi

Tai Chi is a form of martial art that emphasizes slow, controlled movements and deep breathing. It is excellent for improving balance, stability, and overall body awareness.

How to Perform:

- Find a Tai Chi class or follow along with an online video.

- Focus on slow, deliberate movements and maintaining your balance throughout the practice.
- Practice regularly to see improvements in balance and stability.

5. Yoga

Many yoga poses challenge and improve balance while also enhancing flexibility and strength.

Examples of Yoga Poses for Balance:

- **Tree Pose (Vrksasana):** Stand on one leg and place the sole of the other foot on your inner thigh or calf. Hold the pose while focusing on a point in front of you.
- **Warrior III (Virabhadrasana III):** Stand on one leg and extend the other leg behind you while leaning forward, creating a straight line from your head to your extended foot.

Integrating Balance Training into Your Workouts

To reap the full benefits of balance training, it's important to integrate these exercises into your regular workout routine. Here's how you can do it:

1. Warm-Up and Cool-Down

Include balance exercises in your warm-up and cool-down routines. This prepares your body for more intense activities and helps improve overall balance and stability.

Example Warm-Up Routine:

- Start with dynamic stretching and light cardio to increase blood flow.
- Perform single-leg stands, heel-to-toe walks, and balance board exercises.

Example Cool-Down Routine:

- Finish your workout with static stretching and balance exercises.
- Include yoga poses like Tree Pose and Warrior III to enhance flexibility and balance.

2. Balance-Focused Workouts

Dedicate specific workout sessions to balance and stability training. This ensures that you are consistently working on these important aspects of fitness.

Example Balance Workout:

- Warm-up: 5-10 minutes of light cardio and dynamic stretching.
- Balance exercises: Single-leg stands, heel-to-toe walks, balance board exercises, and yoga poses.
- Core strengthening: Planks, side planks, and bridges to enhance core stability.
- Cool-down: Static stretching and deep breathing exercises.

3. Incorporate Balance into Other Workouts

Add balance challenges to your regular strength training and cardio workouts. This can be done by performing exercises on unstable surfaces or adding balance components to traditional exercises.

Examples:

- Perform squats on a Bosu ball or balance board.
- Use a stability ball for exercises like push-ups and planks.
- Add single-leg exercises to your strength training routine, such as single-leg deadlifts and single-leg squats.

4. Progressive Overload

Just like other forms of exercise, balance training should follow the principle of progressive overload. Gradually increase the difficulty of your balance exercises to continue challenging your body and making progress.

Progression Ideas:

- Start with simple exercises like single-leg stands and progress to more challenging ones like single-leg deadlifts.
- Increase the duration of each balance exercise as you improve.
- Use unstable surfaces like balance boards, Bosu balls, or foam pads to add difficulty.

Chapter 8: Proper Form and Technique

Mastering proper form and technique is fundamental for anyone embarking on a fitness journey. Not only does it maximize the effectiveness of your workouts, but it also significantly reduces the risk of injury. This chapter will explore the importance of proper form, common mistakes to avoid, and provide practical tips for maintaining good posture and alignment during various exercises.

The Importance of Proper Form to Prevent Injury

1. **Minimizing the Risk of Injury** Proper form ensures that your body moves in a biomechanically efficient manner, minimizing unnecessary strain on muscles, joints, and connective tissues. Incorrect form can lead to acute injuries like sprains and strains or chronic conditions such as tendonitis and joint pain. By focusing on proper technique, you can perform exercises safely and reduce the likelihood of injury.

2. **Maximizing Workout Effectiveness** Exercising with proper form targets the intended muscle groups more effectively, leading to better results. For instance, performing a squat with proper alignment engages the quadriceps, hamstrings, glutes, and core muscles more effectively than if done with poor form. Proper technique allows for full range of motion, ensuring that each muscle is worked to its potential.

3. **Promoting Muscle Balance and Symmetry** Proper form helps in developing muscle balance

and symmetry. Imbalances often occur when certain muscles compensate for weaker ones, leading to overuse injuries and postural issues. Correct form ensures that all muscles are engaged appropriately, promoting balanced muscle development and preventing compensatory movements.

4. **Building a Solid Foundation** Learning and practicing proper form builds a solid foundation for more advanced exercises and techniques. It establishes good habits early on, making it easier to progress safely and effectively as your fitness level improves. This foundation is crucial for long-term success and sustainability in any fitness program.

Common Mistakes to Avoid During Exercise

1. **Rounding the Back** One of the most common mistakes, especially during exercises like deadlifts and rows, is rounding the back. This places excessive strain on the spine and can lead to serious injuries. Always keep your back straight, chest lifted, and core engaged.

2. **Locking Joints** Locking your knees, elbows, or other joints during exercises can lead to hyperextension and increase the risk of injury. Keep a slight bend in your joints to maintain tension in the muscles and protect the joints.

3. **Using Momentum** Swinging weights or using momentum to lift can compromise form and reduce the effectiveness of the exercise. Focus

on controlled movements, engaging the targeted muscles throughout the entire range of motion.

4. **Incorrect Foot Placement** Incorrect foot placement can affect balance and alignment, particularly in exercises like squats and lunges. Ensure your feet are positioned correctly, typically shoulder-width apart for squats and hip-width apart for lunges, with toes pointing forward or slightly outward.

5. **Overarching the Lower Back** Overarching the lower back, especially during pressing movements like bench presses or overhead presses, can strain the spine. Maintain a neutral spine position by engaging your core and avoiding excessive arching.

6. **Lifting Too Heavy** Using weights that are too heavy can compromise form and increase the risk of injury. Choose a weight that allows you to perform the exercise with proper form and control. Gradually increase the weight as your strength improves.

Tips for Maintaining Good Posture and Alignment

1. **Engage Your Core** A strong, engaged core is essential for maintaining proper alignment and stability during exercises. Practice core activation by drawing your belly button toward your spine and maintaining this engagement throughout your workout.

2. **Check Your Alignment** Regularly check your alignment in a mirror or ask a trainer to provide feedback. Ensure your head, shoulders, hips,

and knees are aligned, and avoid any excessive tilting or shifting.

3. **Use Cues and Visualizations** Using cues and visualizations can help maintain proper form. For example, imagine holding a coin between your shoulder blades during a row to avoid rounding your back, or think about sitting back into a chair during a squat to keep your knees from drifting forward.

4. **Perform Mobility Exercises** Incorporate mobility exercises into your routine to improve your range of motion and flexibility. This helps maintain proper alignment and reduces the risk of compensatory movements due to tight muscles.

5. **Start with Bodyweight Exercises** Before adding weights, master bodyweight exercises to ensure proper form and technique. Exercises like bodyweight squats, push-ups, and planks are excellent for building foundational strength and practicing correct alignment.

6. **Use Proper Breathing Techniques** Proper breathing supports good posture and form. Exhale during the exertion phase of an exercise (e.g., lifting the weight) and inhale during the return phase (e.g., lowering the weight). This helps maintain stability and control throughout the movement.

7. **Warm-Up and Cool-Down** Always warm up before your workout to prepare your muscles and joints for exercise. A proper warm-up increases blood flow, enhances flexibility, and reduces the risk of injury. Similarly, cooling

down with stretching exercises helps maintain flexibility and prevents muscle stiffness.

Practical Application: Common Exercises

1. **Squats**
   - **Form Tips:** Stand with feet shoulder-width apart, toes pointing slightly outward. Keep your chest up, shoulders back, and core engaged. Lower your body by bending your knees and hips, keeping your weight on your heels. Avoid letting your knees go past your toes and maintain a neutral spine.
   - **Common Mistakes:** Knees collapsing inward, heels lifting off the ground, and excessive forward lean.
2. **Push-Ups**
   - **Form Tips:** Start in a plank position with hands shoulder-width apart. Keep your body in a straight line from head to heels. Lower your body by bending your elbows, keeping them close to your sides. Push back up to the starting position.
   - **Common Mistakes:** Sagging hips, flaring elbows, and limited range of motion.
3. **Deadlifts**
   - **Form Tips:** Stand with feet hip-width apart, barbell over mid-foot. Bend at the hips and knees to grasp the bar, keeping your back straight and chest up. Lift the

bar by straightening your hips and knees, maintaining a neutral spine. Lower the bar back to the ground with control.

- o **Common Mistakes:** Rounding the back, lifting with the lower back instead of the legs, and using too much weight.

4. **Planks**

- o **Form Tips:** Start on your hands and knees, then lower your forearms to the ground. Extend your legs back to form a straight line from head to heels. Keep your core tight, avoiding any sagging or lifting of the hips.
- o **Common Mistakes:** Dropping the hips, arching the back, and holding the breath.

5. **Lunges**

- o **Form Tips:** Stand with feet hip-width apart. Step forward with one leg, lowering your hips until both knees are bent at a 90-degree angle. Keep your front knee directly above your ankle and your back knee just above the ground. Push back to the starting position and repeat on the other side.
- o **Common Mistakes:** Allowing the front knee to extend past the toes, leaning forward, and losing balance.

Chapter 9: Injury Prevention and Management

Injury prevention and management are crucial components of any fitness routine, especially for beginners. Understanding how to recognize and prevent common exercise injuries can help you maintain a consistent workout schedule and avoid setbacks. This chapter will delve into the strategies for safe exercising, including the importance of warm-ups and cool-downs, basic first aid, and when to seek professional help.

How to Recognize and Prevent Common Exercise Injuries

1. **Common Exercise Injuries**
   - **Strains and Sprains:** These occur when muscles or ligaments are overstretched or torn. Symptoms include pain, swelling, and reduced range of motion.
   - **Tendinitis:** Inflammation of the tendons often caused by repetitive motion. It presents as pain and tenderness around the affected joint.
   - **Stress Fractures:** Small cracks in the bones due to repetitive force or overuse. They manifest as localized pain that worsens with activity.
   - **Shin Splints:** Pain along the shinbone, commonly caused by overuse or improper footwear.

- o **Runner's Knee:** Pain around the kneecap, often due to improper tracking of the kneecap or muscle imbalances.
- o **Lower Back Pain:** Commonly caused by improper lifting technique, poor posture, or weak core muscles.

2. **Preventing Exercise Injuries**
   - o **Proper Warm-Up:** Warming up increases blood flow to the muscles, enhances flexibility, and prepares your body for the workout ahead. A proper warm-up should last 5-10 minutes and include dynamic stretches and light cardio activities such as jogging or jumping jacks.
   - o **Correct Form and Technique:** Using proper form and technique is crucial to prevent injuries. Focus on maintaining good posture, using controlled movements, and avoiding excessive strain on any particular muscle group.
   - o **Gradual Progression:** Avoid pushing your body too hard too soon. Gradually increase the intensity, duration, and frequency of your workouts to allow your body to adapt.
   - o **Adequate Rest and Recovery:** Ensure you get enough rest between workouts to allow your muscles to repair and grow. Overtraining can lead to fatigue and increase the risk of injury.
   - o **Balanced Workout Routine:** Incorporate a mix of cardiovascular,

strength training, flexibility, and balance exercises to ensure overall fitness and reduce the risk of overuse injuries.

- o **Proper Footwear and Equipment:** Use appropriate footwear and equipment for your chosen activities to provide the necessary support and reduce injury risk.
- o **Listening to Your Body:** Pay attention to any signs of discomfort or pain and adjust your workouts accordingly. Ignoring these signs can lead to more severe injuries.

Tips for Safe Exercising

1. **Warm-Ups**
   - o **Dynamic Stretching:** Perform dynamic stretches such as leg swings, arm circles, and walking lunges to increase flexibility and prepare your muscles for more intense activity.
   - o **Light Cardio:** Engage in light cardio activities like brisk walking, jogging, or cycling to raise your heart rate and improve circulation.
2. **Cool-Downs**
   - o **Static Stretching:** After your workout, perform static stretches to help relax your muscles and improve flexibility. Hold each stretch for 20-30 seconds, focusing on the major muscle groups used during your workout.

- **Gentle Movement:** Engage in gentle movements such as walking or slow cycling to gradually bring your heart rate down to its resting level.

3. **Hydration and Nutrition**
   - **Stay Hydrated:** Drink water before, during, and after your workouts to stay hydrated. Dehydration can lead to muscle cramps, fatigue, and decreased performance.
   - **Balanced Diet:** Consume a balanced diet rich in proteins, carbohydrates, healthy fats, vitamins, and minerals to fuel your workouts and aid recovery.

4. **Proper Breathing Techniques**
   - **Inhale and Exhale:** Focus on your breathing during exercises. Inhale deeply through your nose and exhale through your mouth, coordinating your breath with your movements to maintain stability and control.

5. **Listening to Your Body**
   - **Pain vs. Discomfort:** Learn to differentiate between the discomfort of a challenging workout and the pain of a potential injury. Stop exercising if you experience sharp, shooting, or severe pain and seek medical advice if necessary.
   - **Rest Days:** Incorporate rest days into your routine to allow your body to recover and prevent overtraining.

Basic First Aid and When to Seek Professional Help

1. **Basic First Aid for Common Injuries**
   - **R.I.C.E. Method:** For strains, sprains, and other minor injuries, use the R.I.C.E. method—Rest, Ice, Compression, and Elevation. Rest the injured area, apply ice to reduce swelling, use a compression bandage to support the injury, and elevate the injured limb above heart level.
   - **Heat Therapy:** For muscle soreness and stiffness, apply a heat pack or take a warm bath to relax the muscles and improve blood flow.
   - **Over-the-Counter Pain Relief:** Use over-the-counter pain relief medications such as ibuprofen or acetaminophen to manage pain and inflammation.
2. **When to Seek Professional Help**
   - **Persistent Pain:** If pain persists for more than a few days or worsens despite rest and basic first aid, seek medical advice.
   - **Severe Swelling or Bruising:** Severe swelling, bruising, or difficulty moving the affected area may indicate a more serious injury that requires professional evaluation.
   - **Numbness or Tingling:** Numbness, tingling, or loss of sensation can be a sign of nerve damage and should be addressed by a healthcare professional.

- o **Joint Instability:** If a joint feels unstable or gives way, it could indicate a ligament injury that needs medical attention.
- o **Chronic Conditions:** If you have a chronic condition such as arthritis or a previous injury, consult a healthcare provider or physical therapist for personalized advice on safe exercise practices.

Chapter 10: Listening to Your Body

Embarking on a fitness journey is as much about understanding and respecting your body as it is about following a structured exercise routine. Chapter 10, "Listening to Your Body," provides crucial insights into distinguishing between different types of pain, the significance of rest and recovery, and how to tailor exercises to fit your unique fitness level and needs. Mastering these aspects is essential for creating a sustainable and effective workout regimen, enhancing performance, and preventing injuries.

Understanding the Difference between Good Pain and Bad Pain

1. **Good Pain**
   - **What It Is:** Often described as the "muscle burn" or soreness experienced after a workout, good pain is generally a sign that your muscles are adapting and growing stronger. This type of pain, known as delayed onset muscle soreness (DOMS), occurs as a result of microscopic tears in the muscle fibers during exercise.
   - **Characteristics:** Good pain is typically dull, aching, or tender and emerges 24-48 hours after a workout. It should be felt as an overall sense of muscle fatigue rather than sharp or localized pain. This discomfort is a natural part of the

muscle-building process and usually subsides within a few days.

- o **Managing Good Pain:** Stretching, light activity, and proper hydration can help alleviate good pain. Gentle exercises like walking or yoga can promote blood flow to sore muscles, aiding in recovery.

2. **Bad Pain**

- o **What It Is:** Bad pain is often sharp, sudden, and may feel intense or stabbing. It usually indicates an injury or strain, such as a muscle tear, ligament sprain, or joint issue.
- o **Characteristics:** Bad pain is often localized and may be accompanied by swelling, bruising, or difficulty moving the affected area. It can occur suddenly during an exercise and may persist even when at rest.
- o **Managing Bad Pain:** If you experience bad pain, it is crucial to stop the activity immediately and assess the situation. Applying the R.I.C.E. method (Rest, Ice, Compression, Elevation) can provide initial relief, but seeking professional medical advice is recommended if the pain persists or worsens.

The Importance of Rest and Recovery

1. **Why Rest Is Crucial**

- o **Muscle Repair and Growth:** Rest is a fundamental component of any fitness program, allowing muscles to repair and grow stronger after workouts. During rest periods, the body rebuilds muscle fibers that were broken down during exercise, leading to increased strength and endurance.

- **Prevention of Overtraining:** Overtraining occurs when the body is subjected to excessive exercise without adequate rest. This can lead to fatigue, decreased performance, weakened immune function, and increased risk of injuries. Rest prevents overtraining by providing the body with necessary downtime.
- **Mental and Emotional Well-being:** Regular rest also contributes to mental and emotional health, reducing the risk of burnout and maintaining motivation. Overexertion can lead to exercise fatigue, decreased enthusiasm, and an overall negative outlook on fitness.

2. **How to Incorporate Rest and Recovery**
   - **Scheduled Rest Days:** Plan regular rest days into your weekly routine to allow your muscles and joints time to recover. For most people, one to two rest days per week is adequate, but this can vary based on individual fitness levels and workout intensity.
   - **Active Recovery:** Engage in low-intensity activities on rest days, such as walking, swimming, or stretching.

Active recovery helps to keep the body moving without putting additional strain on it, facilitating faster recovery and improved flexibility.

- o **Sleep and Nutrition:** Ensure you get sufficient, high-quality sleep each night, as it is critical for muscle recovery and overall health. Complement your rest with a balanced diet rich in proteins, vitamins, and minerals to support muscle repair and energy replenishment.

How to Modify Exercises to Fit Your Fitness Level and Needs

1. **Adjusting Intensity and Complexity**
   - o **Beginner Modifications:** Start with simpler, less intense versions of exercises. For instance, if traditional push-ups are too challenging, begin with knee push-ups or wall push-ups. Gradually increase the intensity as your strength and technique improve.
   - o **Progressive Overload:** Apply the principle of progressive overload by slowly increasing the weight, resistance, or duration of your exercises. This method helps to continuously challenge your body while minimizing the risk of injury.
   - o **Exercise Variations:** Use variations of exercises to suit different fitness levels. For example, substitute high-impact

exercises with low-impact alternatives if you're recovering from an injury or have joint concerns.

2. **Customizing Your Workout Routine**
   - **Personalized Plans:** Create workout plans that align with your individual fitness goals and limitations. If you have a specific objective, such as building strength or improving flexibility, tailor your exercises to focus on these areas while considering your current fitness level.
   - **Monitoring Progress:** Regularly assess your progress and adjust your workouts accordingly. If an exercise becomes too easy or too difficult, modify the intensity or technique to ensure continued progress and prevent plateaus.
   - **Listening to Feedback:** Pay close attention to how your body responds to different exercises. If you experience discomfort or notice that an exercise causes pain, modify it or replace it with an alternative that suits your needs better.

Chapter 11: Building a Support System

Embarking on a fitness journey can be exhilarating, but sustaining motivation over time often requires more than just personal resolve. Chapter 11, "Building a Support System," delves into how the presence of friends, family, and fitness communities can play a pivotal role in keeping you motivated and committed to your fitness goals. A strong support system not only encourages you but also holds you accountable, making your fitness journey more enjoyable and effective.

The Role of Friends, Family, and Fitness Communities in Staying Motivated

1. **Friends and Family Support**
   - **Encouragement and Motivation:** Having friends and family who support your fitness goals can be incredibly motivating. Their encouragement can provide the extra push needed to stick with your routine, especially on days when you feel less inclined to exercise.
   - **Shared Activities:** Engaging in fitness-related activities with loved ones, such as hiking, biking, or attending fitness classes together, not only strengthens your bond but also makes working out more enjoyable. This shared experience can create positive associations with exercise and make it a regular part of your life.

- o **Emotional Support:** Friends and family can offer emotional support during challenging times, such as when you're facing a plateau or struggling with motivation. Their belief in your ability to succeed can bolster your own self-confidence and persistence.

2. **Fitness Communities**
   - o **Finding Your Tribe:** Joining a fitness community, whether online or in-person, connects you with like-minded individuals who share your health and wellness goals. These communities provide a sense of belonging and camaraderie, which can be incredibly motivating.
   - o **Group Classes and Events:** Participating in group fitness classes or local fitness events introduces you to new workout routines and keeps you engaged. The social aspect of group activities can create a fun and dynamic environment that encourages regular attendance and enthusiasm.
   - o **Online Forums and Social Media:** Engaging with fitness communities on social media platforms or online forums offers a wealth of resources, from workout tips to inspirational success stories. These platforms can also be a space for sharing your own progress and celebrating achievements with a supportive audience.

Finding a Workout Buddy or Joining a Fitness Group

1. **Workout Buddies**
   - **Mutual Motivation:** Finding a workout buddy can significantly enhance your motivation. When you have someone to exercise with, you are more likely to stick to your routine due to the mutual commitment and encouragement. This partnership can also add a social element to your workouts, making them more enjoyable.
   - **Shared Goals and Accountability:** A workout buddy can help you set and achieve fitness goals. They provide a sense of accountability, ensuring you stay on track and committed to your workouts. Regularly scheduled sessions with a buddy can also create a routine that is harder to break.
   - **Variety and Fun:** Exercising with a buddy can introduce variety into your routine. You can try new activities, challenge each other, and enjoy the process of discovering different workouts together, making the experience more engaging and less monotonous.
2. **Fitness Groups**
   - **Structured Environment:** Joining a fitness group provides a structured environment for exercise, often led by

experienced instructors or trainers. This structure ensures that you are following a well-designed workout plan and receiving professional guidance.

- o **Social Interaction:** Fitness groups offer the opportunity to meet new people and build friendships with individuals who share similar health and fitness goals. This social interaction can enhance your motivation and make attending workouts a more pleasant experience.
- o **Competitive Spirit:** Being part of a fitness group can foster a healthy competitive spirit. Friendly competitions and challenges within the group can drive you to push your limits and achieve better results, while also making your fitness journey more enjoyable.

How to Stay Accountable to Your Fitness Goals

1. **Setting Clear and Achievable Goals**
   - o **SMART Goals:** Define your fitness goals using the SMART criteria—Specific, Measurable, Achievable, Relevant, and Time-bound. Clear goals provide direction and motivation, making it easier to track progress and stay committed.
   - o **Regular Check-ins:** Schedule regular check-ins to assess your progress towards your goals. This can be done through self-assessment, fitness tracking

apps, or with your workout buddy or fitness group.

2. **Tracking Progress**
   - **Journals and Apps:** Keep a fitness journal or use tracking apps to monitor your workouts, progress, and achievements. Documenting your journey helps maintain focus and provides a tangible record of your efforts and successes.
   - **Visual Reminders:** Use visual reminders, such as progress photos or motivational quotes, to keep your goals in sight. These reminders can serve as a constant source of inspiration and help reinforce your commitment.

3. **Rewarding Yourself**
   - **Celebrate Milestones:** Recognize and celebrate your achievements, no matter how small. Rewarding yourself for reaching milestones can boost motivation and reinforce positive behavior.
   - **Positive Reinforcement:** Incorporate positive reinforcement into your routine. Treat yourself to something enjoyable, such as a new workout outfit or a relaxing day off, as a reward for your hard work and dedication.

Chapter 12: Overcoming Obstacles

This chapter addresses the inevitable challenges that arise on your fitness journey and provides practical strategies to navigate these hurdles effectively. Recognizing and addressing these common barriers is crucial for maintaining motivation, achieving your goals, and sustaining a long-term commitment to exercise. Whether you're dealing with time constraints, lack of motivation, or other obstacles, this chapter offers solutions to help you stay on track.

Common Barriers to Exercise and How to Overcome Them

1. **Lack of Time**
   - **Identifying Time Constraints:** One of the most common obstacles to regular exercise is a lack of time. Busy schedules, work commitments, and family responsibilities often make it challenging to fit in workouts.
   - **Creating a Flexible Schedule:** To overcome this barrier, prioritize your fitness routine by incorporating it into your daily schedule. Consider shorter, high-intensity workouts that can be completed in 20-30 minutes. Also, look for opportunities to exercise throughout the day, such as taking brisk walks during breaks or using active commuting options like biking or walking to work.

- o **Utilizing Time-Saving Techniques:** Explore time-efficient workout formats such as circuit training, which combines strength and cardio exercises into a single session. High-Intensity Interval Training (HIIT) is another effective method for achieving significant results in a shorter amount of time.

2. **Lack of Motivation**
   - o **Understanding Motivation Fluctuations:** Motivation can ebb and flow, making it difficult to stay consistent with your fitness routine. Identifying the root causes of low motivation—such as burnout, boredom, or unrealistic expectations—can help address this barrier.
   - o **Setting Achievable Goals:** Break down larger fitness goals into smaller, achievable milestones to maintain motivation and track progress. Celebrate these small victories to boost morale and keep yourself engaged.
   - o **Finding Enjoyable Activities:** Choose exercises and activities that you genuinely enjoy. Whether it's dancing, swimming, or group fitness classes, engaging in activities that you find fun will help sustain your interest and motivation.

3. **Lack of Access to Equipment or Facilities**
   - o **Exploring Alternative Options:** Limited access to gyms or exercise

equipment can be a significant obstacle. In such cases, explore bodyweight exercises, which require minimal or no equipment. Examples include push-ups, squats, and planks.

- o **Utilizing Home-Based Solutions:** Create a home workout space with essential equipment such as resistance bands, dumbbells, or a yoga mat. Online workout videos and fitness apps can also provide guided workouts and routines suitable for home exercise.
- o **Embracing Outdoor Activities:** Take advantage of outdoor spaces for exercise. Activities like running, hiking, or cycling can be effective alternatives to gym workouts and provide a refreshing change of scenery.

4. **Physical Limitations or Health Issues**

- o **Addressing Physical Limitations:** Health issues or physical limitations can impact your ability to engage in certain exercises. Consult with a healthcare professional or a fitness specialist to develop a safe and effective exercise plan tailored to your specific needs and conditions.
- o **Adapting Workouts:** Modify exercises to accommodate physical limitations. For example, if you have joint issues, opt for low-impact exercises such as swimming or using an elliptical machine. Focus on exercises that enhance flexibility,

strength, and mobility while minimizing strain on affected areas.

- o **Monitoring and Adjusting:** Regularly monitor your body's response to exercise and make adjustments as needed. Prioritize exercises that improve overall well-being and seek professional guidance if you experience persistent discomfort or pain.

5. **Lack of Knowledge or Experience**

- o **Educating Yourself:** A lack of knowledge or experience can be a barrier to starting or maintaining an exercise routine. Educate yourself on fitness principles, exercise techniques, and proper form through reputable sources such as books, online resources, or fitness professionals.
- o **Seeking Professional Guidance:** Consider working with a certified personal trainer or fitness coach who can provide personalized guidance, create tailored workout plans, and offer feedback on your form and technique.
- o **Starting Small:** Begin with basic exercises and gradually progress as you build confidence and experience. Learning proper form and technique is essential for maximizing effectiveness and reducing the risk of injury.

6. **Cost Constraints**

- o **Exploring Cost-Effective Options:** Budget constraints can limit access to gyms or fitness classes. Explore cost-effective alternatives such as community fitness programs, online workout resources, or outdoor exercise options that require minimal investment.

- o **Using Free Resources:** Take advantage of free fitness resources, including workout apps, YouTube channels, and fitness blogs. Many of these resources offer high-quality workouts and fitness advice at no cost.
- o **Investing Wisely:** If possible, invest in essential fitness equipment that provides long-term value. Items such as resistance bands, dumbbells, or a yoga mat can support a wide range of exercises and are often cost-effective.

7. **Family and Social Commitments**
   - o **Balancing Commitments:** Family and social commitments can sometimes interfere with your exercise routine. Schedule workouts at times that fit seamlessly into your day and involve family members in physical activities to foster a supportive environment.
   - o **Communicating Needs:** Communicate your fitness goals and needs with family members and seek their support. Establish a routine that accommodates both your exercise and family responsibilities.
   - o **Creating Family Workouts:** Plan family-friendly activities that incorporate

physical exercise, such as group walks, bike rides, or active games. This approach ensures that fitness becomes a shared experience rather than a separate commitment.

Strategies for Staying Motivated When Progress is Slow

Experiencing slow progress in your fitness journey can be discouraging, but it's a common part of the process. Understanding how to stay motivated during these times is crucial for maintaining your commitment and achieving long-term success. Here are comprehensive strategies to help you stay focused and motivated even when progress seems slow.

1. Set Realistic and Achievable Goals

- **Adjust Your Expectations:** Understand that fitness progress isn't always linear. It's essential to set realistic, achievable goals that reflect the natural ebb and flow of progress. If you find that your initial goals are too ambitious, adjust them to more manageable milestones.
- **Break Down Goals:** Divide larger goals into smaller, incremental objectives. This approach allows you to focus on short-term achievements and celebrate small victories along the way, keeping your motivation high.

2. Track and Celebrate Small Wins

- **Document Progress:** Keep a fitness journal or use a tracking app to log your workouts, achievements, and any improvements. Seeing how far you've come, even in small ways, can provide a motivational boost.
- **Celebrate Milestones:** Acknowledge and reward yourself for reaching small milestones. Celebrating these achievements helps reinforce positive behavior and keeps you motivated.

3. Reframe Your Perspective

- **Focus on the Process:** Instead of fixating on the end result, shift your focus to the process and the effort you're putting in. Emphasize the positive habits and routines you're building, rather than just the outcomes.
- **Embrace the Journey:** Recognize that setbacks and slow progress are part of the journey. Embrace these challenges as opportunities for growth and learning rather than as failures.

4. Mix Up Your Routine

- **Variety is Key:** Introduce new exercises, activities, or workout formats to keep things fresh and exciting. Variety not only prevents boredom but can also help overcome plateaus by challenging your body in new ways.
- **Try New Classes or Sports:** Explore different types of workouts, such as group fitness classes, sports, or outdoor activities. Engaging in new

and enjoyable activities can reignite your passion for fitness.

5. Seek Social Support

- **Find a Workout Buddy:** Partnering with a friend, family member, or fitness group can provide encouragement, accountability, and a sense of camaraderie. Sharing your fitness journey with others can make it more enjoyable and less isolating.
- **Join Fitness Communities:** Engage with online or local fitness communities to connect with others who share similar goals. Being part of a supportive group can offer motivation, advice, and inspiration.

6. Reevaluate and Adjust Your Plan

- **Assess Your Strategy:** If progress is slow, it might be time to reassess your workout plan, nutrition, or overall approach. Consider consulting with a fitness professional to adjust your plan for better results.
- **Set New Challenges:** Introducing new challenges or variations in your routine can reinvigorate your interest and push through stagnation. Whether it's increasing weights, trying advanced exercises, or setting a new fitness goal, fresh challenges can stimulate progress.

7. Focus on Non-Scale Victories

- **Measure Progress Differently:** Shift your focus from traditional metrics like weight or performance to other indicators of progress. Consider improvements in energy levels, mood, strength, endurance, or flexibility.
- **Recognize Everyday Benefits:** Pay attention to how exercise enhances your overall quality of life. Better sleep, reduced stress, and improved daily functioning are valuable benefits that contribute to long-term motivation.

8. Maintain a Positive Mindset

- **Practice Self-Compassion:** Be kind to yourself and avoid self-criticism. Understand that slow progress is a natural part of the fitness journey, and it doesn't diminish your efforts or worth.
- **Stay Optimistic:** Cultivate a positive attitude by focusing on the benefits of exercise and the progress you've made. Optimism can help you persevere through challenging times and maintain motivation.

9. Utilize Visualization Techniques

- **Visualize Success:** Regularly visualize your fitness goals and the success you aspire to achieve. Imagining yourself reaching your goals can enhance motivation and reinforce your commitment.
- **Create a Vision Board:** Use a vision board to display images, quotes, and reminders of your fitness goals. Visual cues can serve as powerful

motivators and keep you focused on your objectives.

10. Seek Professional Guidance

- **Work with a Trainer:** Consider working with a personal trainer or coach who can provide personalized guidance, support, and encouragement. A professional can help you adjust your routine and offer strategies to overcome plateaus.
- **Consult with a Nutritionist:** If you suspect that nutrition might be affecting your progress, consult with a nutritionist to ensure you're fueling your body correctly for optimal performance and recovery.

Tips for Maintaining an Exercise Routine During Busy Times

Balancing a busy schedule with a consistent exercise routine can be challenging, but with strategic planning and a few practical adjustments, it's possible to stay committed to your fitness goals even when life gets hectic. Here's an extensive guide with tips to help you maintain your exercise routine amidst a busy lifestyle:

1. Prioritize and Schedule Workouts

- **Treat Exercise Like an Appointment:** Block out specific times in your calendar for workouts as you would for any important meeting or commitment. This helps ensure that exercise becomes a non-negotiable part of your schedule.

- **Plan Ahead:** Dedicate a day each week to plan your workouts and make any necessary adjustments to fit your schedule. Having a plan in place minimizes the likelihood of skipping workouts due to a lack of time.

2. Optimize Your Workout Duration

- **Short but Effective:** Embrace shorter, high-intensity workouts that provide maximum benefits in minimal time. Sessions of 20-30 minutes can be highly effective, especially if they incorporate high-intensity interval training (HIIT) or circuit training.
- **Micro-Workouts:** Break your exercise routine into shorter segments that can be spread throughout the day. For instance, you can do a quick 10-minute workout in the morning, a short walk during lunch, and a few minutes of stretching in the evening.

3. Incorporate Exercise into Daily Activities

- **Active Commuting:** If possible, walk or cycle to work, or park farther away to increase your daily step count. Alternatively, consider using public transportation with built-in walking or biking options.
- **Use Breaks Wisely:** Utilize work breaks or downtime for quick exercises, such as desk

stretches, stair climbing, or brief bodyweight workouts. These small bursts of activity can add up over the day.

4. Multitask with Exercise

- **Combine Activities:** Incorporate exercise into other activities, such as listening to audiobooks or podcasts while walking or exercising. This allows you to make the most of your time while still engaging in activities you enjoy.
- **Family Fitness:** Include your family or household members in your workouts. Activities like family bike rides, playing sports together, or group fitness classes can help you stay active while spending quality time with loved ones.

5. Set Realistic Goals

- **Adjust Expectations:** Recognize that during busy periods, your workout routine might need to be adjusted. Set realistic and flexible goals that accommodate your schedule while still challenging you.
- **Focus on Consistency:** Prioritize consistency over intensity. Even if you can only fit in a shorter or less intense workout, maintaining a regular routine is more beneficial than sporadic, lengthy sessions.

6. Choose Convenient Workout Options

- **Home Workouts:** Opt for home-based workouts that eliminate the need for travel to a gym. Utilize online workout programs, fitness apps, or exercise videos that allow you to work out in the comfort of your home.
- **Minimal Equipment:** Invest in basic, versatile equipment like resistance bands, dumbbells, or a yoga mat that doesn't require much space or setup time. This makes it easier to squeeze in a workout whenever you have a few spare minutes.

7. Create a Motivating Environment

- **Designate a Workout Space:** Set up a dedicated area in your home for exercise. Having a specific space can make it easier to transition into workout mode and reduce excuses for skipping workouts.
- **Visual Reminders:** Place motivational quotes, fitness goals, or progress charts where you can see them. These visual reminders can inspire you to stay committed to your routine.

8. Stay Flexible and Adaptable

- **Modify Your Routine:** Be prepared to adjust your workout routine based on your current schedule. If you can't complete your planned workout, adapt by choosing a shorter or different type of exercise.
- **Embrace Variety:** Incorporate a range of activities that can be done in varying time

frames or locations. This flexibility helps you stay engaged and prevents the routine from becoming monotonous.

9. Leverage Technology

- **Fitness Apps:** Use fitness apps to schedule workouts, set reminders, and track your progress. Many apps offer short, efficient workout programs tailored to busy schedules.
- **Virtual Classes:** Participate in virtual fitness classes or live-streamed workouts that can be done from home or any location. This provides the flexibility to fit in workouts at convenient times.

10. Reward Yourself and Stay Positive

- **Celebrate Achievements:** Acknowledge and reward yourself for sticking to your exercise routine, even during busy times. Small rewards or personal incentives can provide additional motivation.
- **Maintain a Positive Attitude:** Focus on the positive aspects of staying active, such as improved energy levels, reduced stress, and better overall well-being. A positive mindset can help you stay motivated and committed to your fitness goals.

Chapter 13: Celebrating Progress

Tracking Your Fitness Progress

In the journey toward achieving your fitness goals, tracking your progress is a critical component that not only provides motivation but also helps in making informed adjustments to your workout routine. Celebrating progress, no matter how small, reinforces your commitment, builds confidence, and keeps you engaged in your fitness journey. Here's an in-depth guide on how to effectively track your progress and celebrate your achievements:

1. Establish Clear Metrics

- **Define Your Goals:** Start by setting specific, measurable goals that align with your overall fitness objectives. These might include goals related to weight loss, strength gains, endurance improvements, flexibility, or other fitness milestones.
- **Choose Key Performance Indicators (KPIs):** Identify the metrics that will best measure your progress toward these goals. Common KPIs include body measurements (waist, hips, etc.), weight, body fat percentage, endurance levels (e.g., how far you can run), strength (e.g., how much weight you can lift), and flexibility improvements.

2. Use a Fitness Journal

- **Document Your Workouts:** Maintain a fitness journal where you record details of each workout session, including exercises performed, sets, reps, weights, and duration. This helps track your progress over time and spot trends or patterns.
- **Note Your Feelings:** Include personal reflections on how you felt during and after each workout. This qualitative data provides insights into your overall well-being and how different workouts impact your mood and energy levels.

3. Leverage Technology

- **Fitness Apps:** Utilize fitness tracking apps that allow you to log workouts, track progress, and analyze performance trends. Many apps offer features such as workout logs, goal setting, progress charts, and integration with wearable fitness devices.
- **Wearable Devices:** Use fitness trackers or smartwatches to monitor real-time metrics like heart rate, steps taken, calories burned, and sleep patterns. These devices provide valuable data to help you evaluate your progress and make adjustments to your routine.

4. Take Regular Measurements

- **Body Measurements:** Track physical changes by measuring key areas of your body, such as waist, hips, chest, arms, and legs. Regular measurements can highlight changes in body composition and provide tangible evidence of progress.

- **Photos:** Take progress photos from consistent angles under the same lighting conditions. Comparing these photos over time can visually document changes in your physique and provide motivation.

5. Set Up Fitness Assessments

- **Perform Regular Assessments:** Schedule periodic fitness assessments to evaluate your progress. These assessments might include performance tests (e.g., timed runs, strength tests), flexibility evaluations, and body composition analysis.
- **Compare Results:** Analyze assessment results over time to determine improvements in strength, endurance, flexibility, and overall fitness. Use this data to adjust your training regimen and set new goals.

6. Celebrate Milestones

- **Recognize Achievements:** Acknowledge and celebrate significant milestones, such as completing a challenging workout, achieving a new personal best, or reaching a specific goal. Celebrating these moments reinforces your progress and motivates you to continue working toward new objectives.

- **Reward Yourself:** Treat yourself to a reward for achieving milestones. This could be something fitness-related, like new workout gear, or a non-fitness reward, like a relaxing day off. Rewards provide positive reinforcement and keep you motivated.

7. Share Your Success

- **Community Support:** Share your progress with friends, family, or fitness communities. Discussing your achievements and receiving encouragement from others can enhance your motivation and sense of accomplishment.
- **Social Media:** If you're comfortable, share your fitness journey and progress on social media. Documenting your achievements publicly can hold you accountable and inspire others.

8. Reflect and Adjust

- **Evaluate Your Progress:** Regularly reflect on your progress and evaluate what has been effective and what needs adjustment. This reflection helps identify successful strategies and areas for improvement.
- **Adjust Your Goals:** Based on your progress, consider adjusting your goals to ensure they remain challenging and relevant. Setting new goals or refining existing ones keeps you engaged and focused.

9. Maintain a Positive Mindset

- **Embrace Small Wins:** Recognize and celebrate small victories along the way. Even incremental progress is a sign of advancement and should be celebrated.
- **Stay Motivated:** Use tracking and celebrating progress as tools to maintain a positive mindset. Focus on your achievements rather than setbacks and remind yourself of how far you've come.

The Importance of Celebrating Small Victories

1. Reinforcement of Positive Behavior

Celebrating small victories reinforces the positive behaviors and actions that lead to success. When you acknowledge and reward yourself for reaching small milestones, you create a cycle of positive reinforcement that encourages continued effort and persistence. This process strengthens the connection between hard work and reward, making it more likely that you will maintain your motivation and commitment to your goals.

- **Psychological Impact:** Positive reinforcement through celebration boosts your self-esteem and confidence. It helps solidify the belief that you are capable of achieving your goals, which can be particularly valuable during challenging phases of your journey.
- **Behavioral Reinforcement:** Regularly celebrating small successes reinforces the habits and routines that contribute to achieving larger

objectives. This consistent reinforcement builds a strong foundation for long-term success.

2. Sustaining Motivation

Small victories act as motivational fuel that keeps you engaged and driven. They provide a tangible sense of progress, which is crucial for maintaining momentum, especially when the path to your ultimate goal seems long or arduous.

- **Immediate Gratification:** Celebrating small wins provides immediate gratification and a sense of accomplishment. This helps to counteract the frustration that can occur when progress toward larger goals seems slow or distant.
- **Psychological Boost:** Each small victory acts as a boost to your motivation, making it easier to tackle subsequent challenges with renewed energy and enthusiasm.

3. Building Confidence and Self-Efficacy

Recognizing and celebrating small successes builds your confidence and sense of self-efficacy. As you experience and acknowledge these victories, you develop a stronger belief in your ability to achieve your overall goals.

- **Enhanced Confidence:** Each small success enhances your self-confidence, making you more resilient to setbacks and better equipped to handle future challenges.

- **Increased Self-Efficacy:** Celebrating small wins fosters a belief in your capability to effect change and achieve larger goals, thereby increasing your overall self-efficacy and drive.

4. Creating a Positive Feedback Loop

Celebrating small victories creates a positive feedback loop that sustains engagement and enthusiasm for your goals. This loop reinforces the idea that progress, no matter how incremental, is valuable and worth pursuing.

- **Continuous Improvement:** Acknowledging small achievements encourages continuous improvement and adaptability. It fosters a mindset of ongoing growth and progress.
- **Positive Attitude:** By focusing on small wins, you cultivate a positive attitude toward your goals and the process of achieving them. This positive outlook helps to overcome challenges and maintain resilience.

5. Enhancing Goal Achievement

Small victories provide clear markers of progress and success, helping you stay focused and aligned with your goals. They break down larger objectives into manageable steps, making it easier to track progress and make adjustments as needed.

- **Progress Tracking:** Celebrating small milestones allows you to track progress more effectively, providing insights into what

strategies are working and where adjustments may be needed.
- **Goal Clarity:** Regularly achieving and celebrating small goals helps clarify the path toward larger objectives, making it easier to stay on course and adjust your approach as necessary.

6. Boosting Enjoyment and Satisfaction

Acknowledging and celebrating small victories enhances your enjoyment and satisfaction with the process of achieving your goals. It makes the journey more enjoyable and fulfilling, which contributes to a more positive overall experience.

- **Increased Enjoyment:** Recognizing and celebrating successes makes the pursuit of your goals more enjoyable, helping you stay engaged and motivated throughout the journey.
- **Fulfillment:** Celebrating achievements provides a sense of fulfillment and satisfaction, reinforcing the value of your efforts and making the pursuit of your goals more rewarding.

7. Fostering a Growth Mindset

Celebrating small victories fosters a growth mindset by emphasizing progress and learning over perfection. It encourages you to view setbacks and challenges as opportunities for growth rather than failures.

- **Embracing Challenges:** A growth mindset helps you embrace challenges and view them as opportunities for learning and improvement. Celebrating small victories reinforces this perspective.

- **Continuous Learning:** Acknowledging incremental progress encourages a focus on continuous learning and development, rather than solely on achieving end goals.

Setting New Goals and Challenges to Stay Engaged

1. The Role of Goal Setting in Sustaining Engagement

Setting new goals and challenges is a dynamic strategy to keep your motivation high and maintain a sense of purpose throughout your journey. As you progress toward achieving your initial objectives, it's crucial to introduce new goals and challenges to prevent stagnation and ensure continued growth.

- **Dynamic Progression:** Introducing new goals keeps the journey dynamic and engaging. It provides a continuous sense of purpose and direction, ensuring that you remain focused and committed to your long-term success.
- **Avoiding Plateau:** Without new goals, you risk hitting a plateau where progress stalls. Setting fresh challenges helps to overcome these plateaus, ensuring that your progress remains steady and your motivation remains strong.

2. Aligning New Goals with Personal Growth

Setting new goals that align with your personal growth and evolving interests enhances your engagement and satisfaction. As you advance, your capabilities and interests may shift, and your goals should reflect these changes to remain relevant and motivating.

- **Reflecting on Achievements:** Evaluate your previous accomplishments to identify areas for further growth. This reflection helps to align new goals with your evolving strengths and interests.
- **Adapting to Changes:** Your goals should adapt to changes in your life, skills, and aspirations. Setting goals that reflect your current ambitions ensures that you stay engaged and excited about your journey.

3. Types of New Goals and Challenges

To maintain engagement, it's essential to diversify the types of goals and challenges you set. This variety not only keeps the process interesting but also ensures a well-rounded approach to personal development.

- **Short-Term Goals:** These are immediate, actionable targets that provide quick wins and maintain motivation. Examples include mastering a new exercise technique or achieving a personal best in a fitness activity.
- **Long-Term Goals:** These are broader objectives that guide your overall journey. Setting milestones for these goals keeps you

focused on the bigger picture while achieving smaller successes along the way.

- **Skill-Based Challenges:** These challenges involve learning new skills or techniques, such as trying a new workout style or mastering a complex exercise. They keep the process engaging by introducing variety and novelty.
- **Performance-Based Goals:** These involve setting targets related to performance metrics, such as improving endurance, strength, or flexibility. They provide tangible benchmarks to measure progress and maintain motivation.

4. Strategies for Effective Goal Setting

To ensure that your new goals and challenges are effective and motivating, it's important to follow certain strategies and principles.

- **SMART Goals:** Ensure that your goals are Specific, Measurable, Achievable, Relevant, and Time-bound. This framework provides clarity and direction, making it easier to track progress and stay focused.
- **Incremental Challenges:** Gradually increase the difficulty of your goals to match your progress. This incremental approach prevents overwhelm and helps you build confidence as you achieve progressively more challenging objectives.
- **Variety and Innovation:** Incorporate a range of goals and challenges to keep the experience fresh and engaging. Experiment with different

types of goals, such as skill development, performance improvement, and personal milestones.

5. Tracking Progress and Celebrating Achievements

Monitoring your progress and celebrating achievements is crucial for maintaining engagement and motivation. Regularly assessing your progress helps you stay on track and recognize your accomplishments.

- **Progress Tracking:** Use tools such as journals, apps, or fitness trackers to monitor your progress. Regularly review your achievements and adjust your goals as needed to stay aligned with your evolving aspirations.
- **Celebration of Success:** Recognize and celebrate your successes, no matter how small. Celebrating achievements provides positive reinforcement and reinforces the value of setting and pursuing new goals.

6. Overcoming Challenges and Staying Resilient

Setting new goals and challenges may come with obstacles and setbacks. Developing resilience and a proactive mindset helps you navigate these challenges effectively.

- **Resilience Building:** Embrace challenges as opportunities for growth and learning. Cultivate resilience by focusing on solutions, seeking support, and maintaining a positive outlook.

- **Proactive Adjustments:** Be prepared to adjust your goals and strategies based on your progress and any obstacles you encounter. Flexibility and adaptability ensure that you stay engaged and motivated despite setbacks.

7. Seeking Inspiration and Support

Engaging with a supportive community and seeking inspiration can provide additional motivation and encouragement as you set and pursue new goals.

- **Community Engagement:** Join fitness groups, online forums, or social media communities related to your goals. Engaging with others who share similar interests provides support, motivation, and accountability.
- **Inspirational Sources:** Draw inspiration from success stories, motivational content, or mentors. Finding sources of inspiration helps you stay focused and motivated as you set and pursue new challenges.

Part 5: Integrating Fitness into Your Lifestyle

Integrating fitness into your lifestyle is not just about setting aside time for workouts; it's about creating a holistic approach to health and well-being that seamlessly blends exercise with your daily life. This part of the book focuses on making fitness an integral and natural component of your routine, ensuring that it enhances rather than disrupts your overall lifestyle.

Here's a detailed and captivating explanation of how to effectively incorporate fitness into your everyday life.

1. Making Fitness a Daily Habit

To truly integrate fitness into your lifestyle, it's essential to develop consistent habits that make exercise a regular part of your day. This involves creating routines that embed physical activity into your existing schedule.

- **Routine Building:** Establish a regular exercise routine by scheduling workouts at specific times each week. Consistency helps make exercise a natural part of your day, similar to other daily activities like eating or sleeping.
- **Habit Formation:** Use strategies such as habit stacking, where you pair a new fitness habit with an existing routine. For example, perform a quick stretching routine right after brushing your teeth each morning. This technique helps reinforce the new habit by associating it with an already established one.
- **Micro-Workouts:** Incorporate shorter, high-intensity workouts into your day if time is limited. Quick bursts of exercise, such as 10-minute routines, can be highly effective and easier to fit into a busy schedule.

2. Combining Fitness with Daily Activities

Integrating fitness doesn't always mean hitting the gym or dedicating a set time to exercise. It's about finding opportunities to incorporate physical activity into your everyday tasks.

- **Active Commuting:** Opt for walking or cycling instead of driving or taking public transport. If you commute by car, park further away to increase your step count. Use stairs instead of elevators, and consider using a standing desk if you work in an office.
- **Active Breaks:** Take advantage of breaks during your day to engage in physical activity. Stretch, do a quick workout, or take a brisk walk during lunch or work breaks. These short intervals of activity can boost your energy levels and overall well-being.
- **Incorporating Exercise into Family Time:** Engage in physical activities with your family or friends, such as hiking, playing sports, or dancing. This not only makes exercise more enjoyable but also promotes a healthy lifestyle for those around you.

3. Creating a Fitness-Friendly Environment

Your environment plays a crucial role in supporting your fitness goals. By making simple adjustments, you can create a space that encourages regular physical activity.

- **Home Gym Setup:** Designate a space in your home for exercise. Equip it with basic fitness equipment, such as dumbbells, resistance bands, or a yoga mat. Having a dedicated space makes it easier to stick to your routine and reduces the excuses for skipping workouts.

- **Fitness-Enhancing Products:** Invest in products that promote physical activity and comfort, such as a quality pair of workout shoes, supportive activewear, or a fitness tracker. These items can enhance your exercise experience and provide additional motivation.
- **Visual Reminders:** Use visual cues, such as posters or motivational quotes, to keep fitness at the forefront of your mind. Place reminders in prominent areas of your home, such as the refrigerator or bathroom mirror, to reinforce your commitment to staying active.

4. Balancing Fitness with Other Responsibilities

Effective integration of fitness involves balancing exercise with other life responsibilities and commitments. It's about finding harmony between physical activity and work, family, and personal time.

- **Time Management:** Prioritize fitness by scheduling it as you would any other important task. Use time management techniques to allocate specific times for exercise while ensuring it fits with your other responsibilities.
- **Flexible Scheduling:** Adapt your workout schedule based on your day-to-day needs. If you have an unexpected change in plans, adjust your exercise routine accordingly. Flexibility allows you to maintain consistency without feeling overwhelmed.

- **Self-Care Integration:** Incorporate fitness into your self-care routine by using it as a way to manage stress and improve overall well-being. Combine physical activity with other self-care practices, such as mindfulness or relaxation techniques, to create a comprehensive approach to health.

5. Staying Motivated and Accountable

Maintaining motivation and accountability is key to successfully integrating fitness into your lifestyle. By employing various strategies, you can keep yourself engaged and committed to your fitness goals.

- **Tracking Progress:** Use tools such as fitness apps, journals, or wearables to monitor your progress. Tracking your achievements helps you stay motivated and provides a sense of accomplishment.
- **Setting New Challenges:** Regularly update your fitness goals and introduce new challenges to keep things exciting. This can include setting new personal records, trying a different workout style, or participating in fitness events.
- **Accountability Partners:** Find a workout buddy, join a fitness group, or share your goals with friends and family. Having someone to exercise with or report to can provide additional motivation and encouragement.

6. Embracing a Holistic Approach to Wellness

Integrating fitness into your lifestyle also involves embracing a holistic approach to overall wellness, which includes not just physical activity but also mental and emotional health.

- **Mindful Living:** Practice mindfulness and stress management techniques alongside your fitness routine. Incorporating mindfulness into your daily life helps you maintain a balanced perspective and enhances your overall well-being.
- **Healthy Eating:** Complement your exercise routine with balanced nutrition. Focus on a diet rich in whole foods, lean proteins, healthy fats, and complex carbohydrates to support your fitness goals and overall health.
- **Sleep and Recovery:** Prioritize quality sleep and recovery to allow your body to repair and rejuvenate. Adequate rest is crucial for maintaining energy levels, improving performance, and preventing injury.

Chapter 14: Nutrition and Hydration

In this Chapter of *Fitness Fundamentals: A Beginner's Guide to Effective Exercise*, we delve into the crucial role of nutrition and hydration in supporting and enhancing your fitness goals. This chapter underscores how the right dietary choices and proper hydration are integral to achieving optimal performance, recovery, and overall health. Here's a comprehensive and captivating exploration of how nutrition and hydration impact your fitness journey:

The Role of Nutrition in Supporting Fitness Goals

1. Fueling Your Workouts

- **Energy Needs:** Nutrition provides the fuel necessary for effective workouts. Carbohydrates, proteins, and fats are the macronutrients that supply energy, with carbohydrates being the primary source for high-intensity exercise. Understanding how to balance these macronutrients helps ensure you have the energy required to perform well during exercise.

- **Pre-Workout Nutrition:** Eating a balanced meal or snack before exercising can improve performance and endurance. A combination of complex carbohydrates and protein, consumed about 1-2 hours before your workout, helps sustain energy levels and supports muscle function.

- **Post-Workout Nutrition:** After exercise, your body needs nutrients to recover and rebuild. Consuming a meal or snack rich in protein and carbohydrates within 30-60 minutes post-workout helps replenish glycogen stores and repair muscle tissues, enhancing recovery and reducing muscle soreness.

2. Building and Repairing Muscle

- **Protein Intake:** Protein plays a vital role in muscle repair and growth. It provides the building blocks (amino acids) necessary for repairing muscle fibers that are broken down during exercise. Incorporating high-quality protein sources such as lean meats, fish, eggs, dairy products, legumes, and plant-based proteins helps support muscle synthesis and overall strength development.
- **Balancing Macronutrients:** While protein is crucial, a well-rounded diet includes an appropriate balance of all macronutrients. Carbohydrates provide energy, fats are essential for hormone production and cell function, and proteins are vital for muscle repair. Balancing these nutrients ensures your body functions optimally and supports your fitness objectives.

3. Supporting Metabolism and Overall Health

- **Metabolic Function:** Proper nutrition supports a healthy metabolism, which is essential for maintaining energy levels and effectively burning calories. Nutrient-dense foods like fruits, vegetables, whole grains, and lean proteins promote metabolic health and can help manage weight.

- **Micronutrients:** Vitamins and minerals play a critical role in overall health and exercise performance. For instance, calcium and vitamin D are important for bone health, while antioxidants like vitamin C and E help reduce exercise-induced oxidative stress. Ensuring a varied diet rich in micronutrients supports your body's physiological functions and recovery processes.

Hydration: The Key to Optimal Performance

1. Importance of Staying Hydrated

- **Fluid Balance:** Proper hydration is vital for maintaining fluid balance, which affects everything from cardiovascular function to muscle contraction. Dehydration can impair performance, reduce endurance, and increase the risk of injury. Drinking adequate fluids before, during, and after exercise helps keep your body hydrated and functioning efficiently.
- **Hydration Strategies:** The amount of fluid needed can vary based on factors such as exercise intensity, duration, and environmental conditions. General guidelines suggest drinking about 8 ounces of water every 20 minutes during intense activity, and more if exercising in hot or humid conditions.

2. Signs of Dehydration

- **Recognizing Symptoms:** Common signs of dehydration include dark-colored urine, dry mouth, dizziness, fatigue, and reduced sweating. Monitoring these symptoms can help you stay aware of your hydration status and take corrective action if needed.
- **Hydration Tips:** To maintain optimal hydration, incorporate water-rich foods such as fruits and vegetables into your diet. Keep a water bottle handy throughout the day and establish a hydration routine, especially if you engage in regular physical activity.

3. Electrolyte Balance

- **Role of Electrolytes:** Electrolytes like sodium, potassium, and magnesium are essential for fluid balance, nerve function, and muscle contraction. During intense exercise, electrolytes are lost through sweat, and it's important to replenish them to avoid imbalances that can affect performance and health.
- **Replenishing Electrolytes:** Sports drinks and electrolyte supplements can help replenish lost electrolytes during prolonged or high-intensity exercise. However, for most people, a balanced diet with foods such as bananas, nuts, and dairy products can provide adequate electrolyte levels.

Creating a Balanced Nutrition Plan

1. Tailoring Your Diet

- **Individual Needs:** Nutrition needs can vary based on factors such as age, gender, fitness level, and specific goals. Tailoring your diet to meet these needs ensures that you get the right nutrients in the appropriate amounts to support your fitness journey.
- **Consulting Professionals:** Working with a registered dietitian or nutritionist can help you develop a personalized nutrition plan that aligns with your fitness goals, dietary preferences, and any specific health considerations.

2. Practical Tips for Healthy Eating

- **Meal Planning:** Plan your meals and snacks to include a variety of nutrient-dense foods. Preparing meals in advance and making healthier choices at home can help you stay on track with your nutrition goals.
- **Mindful Eating:** Practice mindful eating by paying attention to hunger and fullness cues. Eating slowly and savoring your food can help improve digestion and prevent overeating.

Basic Guidelines for a Balanced Diet

A balanced diet is fundamental to achieving optimal health, supporting physical fitness, and enhancing overall well-being. It involves consuming a variety of foods in the right proportions to provide your body with essential nutrients. Here's a comprehensive and detailed look at the key guidelines for maintaining a balanced diet:

1. Macronutrient Distribution

1.1 Carbohydrates

- **Role:** Carbohydrates are the primary source of energy for your body, especially during physical activity. They are broken down into glucose, which fuels your muscles and brain.
- **Sources:** Opt for complex carbohydrates such as whole grains (brown rice, quinoa, oats), vegetables, fruits, and legumes. These provide sustained energy and are rich in fiber, which aids digestion and helps maintain steady blood sugar levels.
- **Portion:** Carbohydrates should constitute about 45-65% of your total daily caloric intake. Balance your carbs with proteins and fats to maintain energy levels and avoid blood sugar spikes.

1.2 Proteins

- **Role:** Proteins are crucial for muscle repair, immune function, and overall cellular health. They provide amino acids that are the building blocks for tissues and enzymes.
- **Sources:** Include a variety of protein sources such as lean meats (chicken, turkey), fish, eggs, dairy products (milk, cheese, yogurt), legumes (beans, lentils), and plant-based proteins (tofu, tempeh).

127

- **Portion:** Proteins should make up about 10-35% of your daily caloric intake. For those engaging in regular exercise or strength training, slightly higher protein intake may be beneficial.

1.3 Fats

- **Role:** Fats are essential for hormone production, cell membrane integrity, and absorbing fat-soluble vitamins (A, D, E, K). They also provide long-term energy storage.
- **Sources:** Focus on healthy fats from sources such as avocados, nuts, seeds, olive oil, and fatty fish (salmon, mackerel). Limit saturated fats found in red meats and processed foods, and avoid trans fats often present in fried and baked goods.
- **Portion:** Fats should comprise about 20-35% of your daily caloric intake. Aim for a balance between unsaturated fats and minimal intake of saturated and trans fats.

2. Micronutrient Intake

2.1 Vitamins

- **Role:** Vitamins are crucial for various bodily functions, including immune support, energy production, and bone health.
- **Sources:** Consume a wide range of fruits and vegetables to ensure you get a diverse array of vitamins. For instance, citrus fruits are rich in

vitamin C, while leafy greens provide vitamin K.

2.2 Minerals

- **Role:** Minerals like calcium, potassium, and iron are vital for bone health, muscle function, and oxygen transport in the blood.
- **Sources:** Dairy products, leafy greens, nuts, seeds, and fortified cereals are good sources of essential minerals. For example, dairy products are high in calcium, while red meat and legumes provide iron.

3. Hydration

3.1 Importance of Water

- **Role:** Water is essential for maintaining hydration, aiding digestion, regulating body temperature, and transporting nutrients.
- **Guideline:** Aim to drink at least 8 glasses (about 2 liters) of water daily, adjusting for activity levels and climate conditions. Increase intake if you're exercising intensely or in hot environments.

3.2 Monitoring Hydration

- **Indicators:** Pay attention to signs of dehydration such as dark urine, dry mouth, or fatigue. Hydrate consistently throughout the day, rather than consuming large amounts in one sitting.

4. Portion Control

4.1 Serving Sizes

- **Guideline:** Be mindful of portion sizes to avoid overeating. Use smaller plates and bowls to help regulate portions and practice mindful eating.
- **Examples:** A standard serving of protein should be about the size of a deck of cards, while a serving of vegetables should cover half your plate.

4.2 Balanced Meals

- **Composition:** Each meal should ideally include a mix of protein, carbohydrates, and healthy fats. For example, a balanced plate might consist of grilled chicken (protein), quinoa (carbohydrate), and a side of roasted vegetables (fiber and nutrients).

5. Dietary Variety

5.1 Incorporating Different Foods

- **Role:** Eating a wide range of foods ensures you get all essential nutrients and minimizes the risk of deficiencies. It also makes your diet more enjoyable and interesting.
- **Strategy:** Rotate different fruits, vegetables, whole grains, and protein sources throughout the week. Experiment with new recipes and cuisines to keep meals exciting and nutritious.

5.2 Avoiding Monotony

- **Avoid:** Relying too heavily on a limited number of foods can lead to nutrient imbalances. Incorporate a variety of foods to ensure comprehensive nutrient intake.

6. Moderation and Balance

6.1 Treats and Indulgences

- **Approach:** While maintaining a balanced diet is important, occasional treats are part of a healthy lifestyle. The key is moderation rather than complete deprivation.
- **Strategy:** Enjoy occasional indulgences in smaller portions, and balance them with healthier choices throughout the day.

6.2 Overall Balance

- **Guideline:** Strive for a balance between different food groups and nutrients. Focus on whole, minimally processed foods while allowing for flexibility and enjoyment in your eating habits.

The Importance of Staying Hydrated Before, During, and After Exercise

Hydration plays a crucial role in optimizing exercise performance, maintaining health, and promoting recovery. Proper hydration before, during, and after exercise is essential for sustaining physical activity, enhancing endurance, and ensuring overall well-being. Here's an in-depth look at why hydration is so important and how to manage it effectively throughout your fitness routine:

1. Hydration Before Exercise

1.1 Preparing the Body

- **Role:** Hydrating before exercise ensures that your body is well-prepared for the physical demands of the workout. Proper hydration helps to maintain blood volume, regulate body temperature, and support cardiovascular function.
- **Guideline:** Aim to drink about 16-20 ounces (500-600 ml) of water at least 2-3 hours before exercise. This helps to ensure that your body is fully hydrated and allows time for excess fluid to be excreted if necessary.

1.2 Benefits for Performance

- **Energy Levels:** Adequate hydration before exercise helps prevent fatigue and enhances energy levels. Dehydration can lead to decreased strength, endurance, and overall performance.
- **Mental Focus:** Being well-hydrated improves cognitive functions, including concentration and reaction times, which are crucial for performance and safety during exercise.

1.3 Avoiding Overhydration

- **Balance:** While it's important to hydrate before exercise, overhydration can also be a concern. Drinking excessive amounts of water in a short period can lead to a condition known as hyponatremia, where sodium levels in the blood become dangerously low. Aim for a balanced approach to hydration.

2. Hydration During Exercise

2.1 Maintaining Fluid Balance

- **Role:** During exercise, especially prolonged or intense workouts, your body loses fluids through sweat and respiration. Drinking fluids helps to maintain optimal fluid balance, prevent dehydration, and sustain performance.
- **Guideline:** For workouts lasting less than an hour, water is typically sufficient. For longer sessions or high-intensity workouts, consider sports drinks that contain electrolytes to replenish lost sodium, potassium, and other minerals.

2.2 Enhancing Performance

- **Prevention of Dehydration:** Regular fluid intake during exercise helps prevent dehydration, which can lead to decreased endurance, increased heart rate, and impaired performance.
- **Temperature Regulation:** Hydration aids in regulating body temperature by enabling efficient sweating and evaporative cooling. This

is particularly important in hot and humid conditions where the risk of heat-related illnesses is higher.

2.3 Practical Tips

- **Sip Regularly:** Aim to drink 7-10 ounces (200-300 ml) of water every 10-20 minutes during exercise. This helps to maintain hydration without overwhelming the digestive system.
- **Monitor Hydration Status:** Pay attention to signs of dehydration such as dark urine, dizziness, or dry mouth. Adjust fluid intake based on these indicators.

3. Hydration After Exercise

3.1 Replenishing Lost Fluids

- **Role:** After exercise, it's essential to replenish fluids lost through sweating and ensure that hydration levels are restored to support recovery. This helps to restore normal bodily functions and prevent dehydration-related symptoms.
- **Guideline:** Drink at least 16-24 ounces (500-750 ml) of water for every pound (0.5 kg) of body weight lost during exercise. This helps to quickly replace lost fluids and supports effective recovery.

3.2 Supporting Recovery

- **Electrolyte Balance:** In addition to water, consider beverages or foods containing electrolytes (sodium, potassium, magnesium) to help restore electrolyte balance, especially after prolonged or intense exercise.
- **Muscle Recovery:** Proper hydration aids in muscle recovery by facilitating nutrient transport to muscle cells and reducing the risk of cramping. It also helps in reducing muscle soreness and fatigue.

3.3 Long-Term Hydration Strategy

- **Consistency:** Hydration should be part of your overall wellness strategy, not just focused on exercise. Maintain good hydration habits throughout the day by drinking water regularly and adjusting intake based on activity level, climate, and personal needs.

3.4 Monitoring Hydration Status

- **Indicators:** Continue to monitor urine color and frequency to gauge hydration levels. Clear or light-colored urine generally indicates adequate hydration, while dark urine can signal the need for increased fluid intake.

Chapter 15: Lifestyle Tips for Staying Active

Maintaining an active lifestyle is essential for long-term health, well-being, and overall quality of life. This chapter delves into practical and motivational strategies to help you integrate physical activity seamlessly into your daily routine. By adopting these lifestyle tips, you can cultivate a habit of staying active, even amidst the demands of a busy life.

1. Incorporating Movement into Daily Routines

1.1 Active Commuting

- **Role:** Transforming your commute into an opportunity for physical activity can significantly increase your daily exercise. Consider walking or cycling to work or using public transport with a walk or bike ride as part of your journey.
- **Benefits:** Active commuting helps build cardiovascular endurance, reduces stress, and integrates exercise into your routine without requiring extra time.

1.2 Household Chores

- **Role:** Everyday chores such as cleaning, gardening, and home maintenance can be excellent sources of physical activity. Engage in these tasks with vigor to maximize their fitness benefits.

- **Examples:** Vacuuming, sweeping, and gardening can provide cardiovascular benefits, while activities like washing windows or carrying groceries can contribute to muscle strength and endurance.

1.3 Standing and Moving at Work

- **Role:** Prolonged sitting can negatively impact health, but incorporating movement into your workday can counteract these effects.
- **Strategies:** Use a standing desk, take regular breaks to stretch or walk, and consider desk exercises or standing meetings to keep active throughout the day.

2. Finding Enjoyable Activities

2.1 Exploring New Hobbies

- **Role:** Engaging in physical activities that you enjoy makes exercise feel less like a chore and more like a fun part of your life.
- **Examples:** Try new activities such as dance classes, hiking, swimming, or team sports. Exploring different options can help you discover what you love and keep your routine exciting.

2.2 Social Engagement

- **Role:** Incorporating social elements into your physical activities can boost motivation and adherence.

- **Strategies:** Join a fitness group, participate in sports leagues, or find a workout buddy. Exercising with friends or in a group setting provides social support and accountability, making it easier to stick with your goals.

3. Setting Realistic and Sustainable Goals

3.1 Goal Setting

- **Role:** Establishing clear and achievable fitness goals helps maintain motivation and provides direction for your activities.
- **SMART Goals:** Use the SMART framework (Specific, Measurable, Achievable, Relevant, Time-bound) to set realistic fitness goals, such as completing a 5K run, attending three workout classes a week, or mastering a new exercise routine.

3.2 Tracking Progress

- **Role:** Regularly tracking your progress helps you stay motivated and see the fruits of your efforts.
- **Methods:** Use fitness apps, journals, or wearable devices to monitor your workouts, progress, and achievements. Celebrating milestones, no matter how small, reinforces positive behaviors and keeps you engaged.

4. Making Exercise a Family Affair

4.1 Family Activities

- **Role:** Including family members in physical activities fosters a supportive environment and promotes healthy habits for everyone.
- **Examples:** Plan family outings that involve physical activity, such as hiking, biking, or playing sports. Engage in home-based activities like family yoga or dance parties to combine fitness with fun.

4.2 Setting Family Fitness Goals

- **Role:** Working towards shared fitness goals can enhance motivation and provide a sense of unity.
- **Strategies:** Set collective goals, such as a family step count challenge or a weekend hike, and encourage each other to stay active. Celebrate achievements together to strengthen bonds and reinforce positive habits.

5. Prioritizing Active Leisure Time

5.1 Active Leisure Activities

- **Role:** Choosing leisure activities that incorporate physical movement helps you stay active while enjoying your free time.
- **Examples:** Opt for active hobbies such as playing sports, hiking, or taking dance classes. These activities not only provide exercise but also offer opportunities for relaxation and enjoyment.

5.2 Balancing Rest and Activity

- **Role:** Balancing periods of rest with active leisure ensures that you stay engaged without overexerting yourself.
- **Strategies:** Incorporate active rest days where you participate in light activities like walking or stretching, rather than complete inactivity. This balance helps maintain your fitness level and promotes overall well-being.

6. Building a Routine

6.1 Establishing Consistency

- **Role:** Creating a consistent exercise routine makes staying active a natural part of your daily life.
- **Tips:** Schedule workouts at times that fit your lifestyle, such as early mornings or after work, and treat them as non-negotiable appointments. Consistency helps form habits and makes physical activity a regular part of your routine.

6.2 Flexibility and Adaptability

- **Role:** Being flexible with your exercise routine allows you to adapt to life's changes and challenges without compromising your fitness goals.
- **Strategies:** Have a range of activities and options available, such as indoor workouts for bad weather or shorter workouts during busy periods. Adapt your routine as needed while maintaining overall activity levels.

Incorporating Physical Activity into Your Daily Routine

Integrating physical activity into your daily routine is key to maintaining a healthy lifestyle and achieving long-term fitness goals. The challenge for many is finding ways to make exercise a regular part of their busy schedules. This detailed guide explores practical strategies and creative solutions to seamlessly incorporate physical activity into your daily life, ensuring that fitness becomes a natural and enjoyable aspect of your routine.

1. Active Commuting

1.1 Transform Your Commute

- **Walking or Cycling:** If feasible, consider walking or cycling to work or school. These activities not only provide cardiovascular benefits but also help you start and end your day on a positive note.
- **Public Transport with Movement:** Use public transportation but add a walk or bike ride as part of your journey. For instance, get off a stop early or park further from your destination to increase your daily steps.

1.2 Utilize Commute Breaks

- **Stretching and Light Exercises:** Use breaks during your commute for stretching or quick exercises. Simple stretches or bodyweight exercises at bus or train stations can help alleviate stiffness and keep you active.

2. Incorporating Activity into Work

2.1 Active Desk Solutions

- **Standing Desks:** Invest in a standing desk or a convertible desk that allows you to alternate between sitting and standing. Standing while working helps reduce the risks associated with prolonged sitting and encourages better posture.
- **Desk Exercises:** Perform desk exercises such as seated leg lifts, chair squats, or shoulder shrugs. These exercises can be done during breaks or while working, contributing to overall physical activity without requiring extra time.

2.2 Regular Movement Breaks

- **Scheduled Breaks:** Set reminders to take short breaks throughout the workday. Use these breaks for quick walks, stretching, or simple exercises. This habit helps combat the negative effects of extended sitting and maintains your activity level.

3. Active Household Chores

3.1 Engage in Vigorous Chores

- **Cleaning:** Approach household cleaning tasks with increased intensity. Vacuuming, mopping, and scrubbing floors can be vigorous activities that raise your heart rate and burn calories.

- **Gardening and Maintenance:** Gardening, yard work, and home maintenance are excellent ways to stay active. These activities involve various muscle groups and contribute to overall physical fitness.

3.2 Incorporate Exercise into Chores

- **Task Modification:** Modify household chores to include exercise. For example, perform squats while picking up laundry or use lunges while carrying groceries. Integrating fitness into daily tasks helps you stay active without needing additional workout time.

4. Family and Social Activities

4.1 Active Family Time

- **Family Outings:** Plan family outings that involve physical activity, such as hiking, biking, or playing sports. Engaging in active leisure with family members not only benefits your health but also strengthens family bonds.
- **Active Games:** Incorporate active games into family gatherings, such as tag, frisbee, or relay races. These activities are fun and provide physical exercise for all ages.

4.2 Social Exercise

- **Workout Buddies:** Find a workout buddy or join a fitness group to add a social element to your exercise routine. Exercising with others can enhance motivation, provide accountability, and make workouts more enjoyable.
- **Group Classes:** Participate in group fitness classes or team sports. Group settings offer social interaction and can help keep you committed to regular physical activity.

5. Fitness Integration into Leisure Time

5.1 Active Leisure Activities

- **Recreational Sports:** Engage in recreational sports such as tennis, basketball, or swimming. These activities provide a fun way to stay active while enjoying your leisure time.
- **Active Hobbies:** Explore hobbies that involve physical movement, such as dancing, rock climbing, or kayaking. Choosing active hobbies ensures that you stay fit while pursuing activities you enjoy.

5.2 Movement During Downtime

- **Active Entertainment:** Opt for active forms of entertainment, such as taking dance classes, joining a sports league, or participating in community fitness events. These activities keep you moving while providing entertainment and social interaction.

6. Flexibility and Adaptability

6.1 Adapting to Busy Schedules

- **Short Workouts:** Incorporate short, high-intensity workouts into your schedule if you have limited time. Even brief sessions of exercise can be effective when done consistently.
- **Exercise Snacking:** Spread physical activity throughout the day by performing short bursts of exercise, such as quick walks, stair climbing, or bodyweight exercises. This approach helps integrate movement into a busy lifestyle.

6.2 Creating Routine Variability

- **Varied Activities:** Keep your routine fresh by varying your activities. This approach prevents boredom and helps you stay motivated. Rotate between different types of exercise, such as cardio, strength training, and flexibility work.
- **Adaptability:** Be flexible with your workout plans and adapt them to fit changes in your schedule or circumstances. Having a range of exercise options allows you to maintain activity levels even when life becomes unpredictable.

Tips for Staying Active at Work and Home

Maintaining physical activity amid the demands of work and home life can be challenging but is essential for overall health and well-being. Balancing productivity with physical fitness requires creativity and deliberate effort. Here's an extensive guide with practical tips to help you stay active at work and home, ensuring that exercise becomes a natural and integrated part of your daily routine.

Staying Active at Work

1. Create an Active Workspace

- **Standing Desks:** Invest in a standing desk or a desk converter that allows you to alternate between sitting and standing. Standing while working reduces the risks associated with prolonged sitting and encourages better posture. Some models come with built-in treadmill options for walking while working.
- **Desk Exercises:** Incorporate desk exercises into your routine, such as seated leg lifts, chair squats, or desk push-ups. These exercises can be performed during short breaks to keep your muscles engaged and your blood flowing.

2. Incorporate Movement Breaks

- **Scheduled Breaks:** Set reminders to take short, frequent breaks throughout the day. Use these breaks for quick walks around the office, stretching, or light exercises. This habit not only combats the negative effects of sitting but also enhances focus and productivity.
- **Active Meetings:** Suggest standing or walking meetings when possible. Standing or walking while discussing work can increase energy levels and foster more dynamic conversations.

3. Use Office Amenities

- **Stair Climbing:** Opt for stairs instead of elevators whenever possible. Climbing stairs is an excellent cardiovascular workout and helps strengthen your leg muscles.
- **Office Fitness Challenges:** Organize or participate in office fitness challenges or wellness programs. Activities like step challenges or fitness competitions can foster a supportive environment and motivate you to stay active.

4. Enhance Your Commute

- **Active Commuting:** If feasible, walk or cycle to work. This not only provides cardiovascular benefits but also serves as a productive start and end to your workday.
- **Public Transport:** Use public transportation but incorporate a walk or bike ride as part of your journey. For example, get off a stop early or park farther away from your destination to increase your daily steps.

Staying Active at Home

1. Integrate Exercise into Daily Chores

- **Vigorous Cleaning:** Approach household cleaning tasks with increased intensity. Activities like vacuuming, mopping, and scrubbing can be vigorous and help you stay active.
- **Active Gardening:** Engage in gardening and yard work, which are physically demanding

activities that also provide a sense of accomplishment and connection with nature.

2. Establish a Home Workout Routine

- **Create a Dedicated Space:** Set up a home exercise area with minimal distractions. Having a dedicated space for workouts makes it easier to stick to your fitness routine.
- **Bodyweight Exercises:** Incorporate bodyweight exercises such as push-ups, squats, lunges, and planks into your daily routine. These exercises require no equipment and can be performed in short sessions throughout the day.

3. Incorporate Movement During Leisure Time

- **Active Hobbies:** Choose hobbies that involve physical movement, such as dancing, hiking, or playing sports. Active hobbies ensure that fitness is enjoyable and naturally integrated into your lifestyle.
- **Family Activities:** Plan family outings that involve physical activity, such as bike rides, hikes, or playing games in the park. Engaging in active leisure with family members not only benefits your health but also strengthens family bonds.

4. Use Technology to Your Advantage

- **Fitness Apps:** Utilize fitness apps or online workout programs that offer guidance and motivation. Many apps provide customizable workout plans and track your progress.

- **Online Classes:** Participate in online fitness classes or virtual group workouts. These classes offer structure and variety, making it easier to stay consistent with your exercise routine.

5. Practice Active Rest

- **Breaks for Movement:** Use breaks to perform quick exercises, such as stretching, yoga poses, or a few minutes of high-intensity interval training (HIIT). Even short bursts of activity can contribute to your overall fitness.
- **Play with Pets:** Engage in active play with pets. Activities like fetch or tug-of-war provide physical exercise for both you and your furry friends.

Maintaining Flexibility and Adaptability

1. Adapt to Changing Schedules

- **Flexible Workouts:** Be adaptable with your exercise routine. If unexpected changes in your schedule occur, adjust your workouts by performing shorter or modified versions of your planned exercises.
- **Exercise Snacking:** Spread physical activity throughout the day with short, high-intensity bursts of exercise. This approach helps maintain your activity level even with a busy schedule.

2. Prioritize Consistency

- **Set Realistic Goals:** Establish achievable fitness goals and integrate them into your daily routine. Consistency is more important than intensity, especially when trying to balance work and home life.
- **Build Habits:** Develop habits that make staying active a natural part of your day. For instance, incorporate exercise into your morning routine or use evening relaxation time for stretching or yoga.

Incorporating physical activity into your work and home life is achievable with thoughtful planning and creativity. By optimizing your workspace, integrating movement into daily chores, leveraging technology, and remaining flexible, you can make exercise a seamless part of your lifestyle. These strategies not only improve your physical health but also enhance your overall well-being, making fitness an integral and enjoyable aspect of your daily routine.

The Benefits of Active Hobbies and Recreational Activities

Incorporating active hobbies and recreational activities into your lifestyle can transform your overall well-being, providing a wealth of physical, mental, and emotional benefits. Engaging in activities that require physical movement not only enhances fitness but also enriches your life in various ways. Here's an extensive exploration of the benefits of active hobbies and recreational activities:

Physical Benefits

1. Improved Cardiovascular Health

Active hobbies, such as dancing, hiking, or playing sports, significantly enhance cardiovascular fitness. These activities elevate your heart rate, which strengthens the heart muscle, improves circulation, and reduces the risk of heart disease. Regular participation in cardiovascular activities helps to maintain healthy blood pressure and cholesterol levels.

2. Increased Muscle Strength and Flexibility

Recreational activities that involve resistance or bodyweight exercises, such as climbing, martial arts, or swimming, contribute to improved muscle strength and flexibility. Building muscle strength through these hobbies supports joint stability and helps prevent injuries. Flexibility exercises, often integrated into activities like yoga or gymnastics, enhance range of motion and reduce muscle stiffness.

3. Weight Management

Active hobbies play a crucial role in managing and maintaining a healthy weight. Activities like cycling, running, or playing tennis burn calories and boost metabolism, aiding in weight loss and preventing obesity. Engaging in regular recreational exercise helps balance energy expenditure with caloric intake, promoting overall weight control.

4. Enhanced Bone Health

Weight-bearing and resistance activities, such as hiking or strength training sports, are beneficial for bone health. These activities stimulate bone density and strength, reducing the risk of osteoporosis and fractures. Active hobbies support bone development and maintenance, particularly important as you age.

Mental Benefits

1. Stress Reduction

Participating in active hobbies provides a natural outlet for stress relief. Physical activity triggers the release of endorphins, which are known as "feel-good" hormones. This chemical reaction helps reduce stress, alleviate anxiety, and improve mood. Engaging in enjoyable activities can also serve as a mental escape from daily pressures and challenges.

2. Improved Cognitive Function

Active hobbies, particularly those requiring coordination and strategy, such as playing sports or learning a new dance routine, enhance cognitive function. These activities stimulate brain activity, improve memory, and boost problem-solving skills. Engaging in complex tasks during recreational activities promotes mental agility and cognitive health.

3. Enhanced Sleep Quality

Regular participation in active hobbies helps regulate sleep patterns and improve sleep quality. Physical activity promotes the production of sleep-inducing hormones and helps establish a regular sleep-wake cycle. Engaging in moderate exercise can lead to deeper, more restorative sleep, reducing insomnia and sleep disturbances.

Emotional Benefits

1. Boosted Self-Esteem and Confidence

Achieving personal goals through active hobbies, such as mastering a new sport or completing a challenging hike, enhances self-esteem and confidence. The sense of accomplishment and progress from these activities reinforces a positive self-image and fosters a greater sense of self-worth.

2. Improved Social Connections

Active hobbies often provide opportunities to connect with others, whether through team sports, fitness classes, or group recreational activities. Building social networks through shared interests promotes a sense of community and belonging. These connections contribute to emotional well-being and provide support systems that enhance overall happiness.

3. Enhanced Mood and Emotional Resilience

Regular involvement in enjoyable recreational activities helps stabilize mood and build emotional resilience. The positive experiences and satisfaction derived from hobbies serve as emotional buffers, helping to cope with life's ups and downs. Engaging in these activities encourages a positive outlook and contributes to emotional stability.

Lifestyle Integration

1. Encouragement of a Balanced Lifestyle

Active hobbies promote a balanced lifestyle by incorporating physical activity into daily routines. Engaging in activities you love, such as gardening, playing sports, or dancing, helps ensure that exercise becomes a natural and enjoyable part of your life. This integration supports long-term commitment to physical health and wellness.

2. Development of Healthy Habits

Regular participation in active hobbies fosters the development of healthy habits. These activities encourage routine exercise and make physical movement an integral part of daily life. By establishing consistent patterns of activity, you build a foundation for ongoing health and fitness.

3. Enhanced Quality of Life

Incorporating active hobbies into your life enriches your overall quality of life. The physical, mental, and emotional benefits collectively contribute to a more fulfilling and vibrant existence. Engaging in recreational activities enhances enjoyment, provides purpose, and adds vitality to daily living.

Active hobbies and recreational activities offer multifaceted benefits that enhance physical health, mental well-being, and emotional stability. By incorporating these activities into your routine, you not only improve your fitness but also enrich your life in numerous ways. Embrace the joy of movement and the positive impact it can have on every aspect of your well-being.

Chapter 16: Mindset and Mental Health

The Connection Between Exercise and Mental Well-Being

Exercise is widely recognized for its physical benefits, but its profound impact on mental health is equally important. This chapter delves into the intricate relationship between physical activity and mental well-being, exploring how exercise can enhance your mental health and overall quality of life. Understanding this connection can motivate you to maintain a consistent exercise routine and prioritize both your physical and mental health.

1. Exercise as a Natural Mood Booster

Endorphin Release

When you engage in physical activity, your body releases endorphins, often referred to as "feel-good" hormones. These natural chemicals interact with receptors in your brain to reduce pain perception and trigger positive feelings. This endorphin rush is commonly known as the "runner's high," but it can be experienced through various forms of exercise, from a brisk walk to an intense workout session. The immediate boost in mood following exercise is a testament to its powerful impact on mental well-being.

Reduction in Stress Hormones

Exercise also plays a crucial role in reducing the levels of stress hormones, such as cortisol and adrenaline. Chronic stress can lead to a range of mental health issues, including anxiety and depression. By regularly engaging in physical activity, you can lower these stress hormone levels, thereby reducing overall stress and promoting a calmer, more balanced state of mind.

2. Enhancing Cognitive Function

Improved Memory and Learning

Exercise has been shown to enhance cognitive functions, including memory and learning. Physical activity increases blood flow to the brain, promoting the growth of new brain cells and improving brain plasticity. This process is particularly beneficial for areas of the brain associated with memory and learning, such as the hippocampus. Regular exercise can improve your ability to learn new information, retain memories, and perform complex cognitive tasks.

Increased Focus and Concentration

Exercise can also boost your ability to focus and concentrate. Physical activity stimulates the production of neurotransmitters like dopamine and norepinephrine, which play a key role in attention and concentration. As a result, individuals who exercise regularly often experience improved productivity, sharper focus, and enhanced problem-solving skills. This cognitive boost is beneficial in both professional and personal aspects of life.

3. Reducing Symptoms of Anxiety and Depression

Natural Anxiety Relief

Exercise is a natural and effective way to alleviate symptoms of anxiety. Physical activity increases the production of neurochemicals that combat anxiety, such as serotonin and gamma-aminobutyric acid (GABA). These chemicals help regulate mood and promote a sense of calm. Additionally, the repetitive nature of many forms of exercise, such as running or cycling, can have a meditative effect, helping to quiet a racing mind and reduce anxiety levels.

Combatting Depression

Exercise has been extensively studied for its ability to reduce symptoms of depression. Regular physical activity can be as effective as medication or psychotherapy for some individuals. Exercise promotes the release of brain-derived neurotrophic factor (BDNF), a protein that supports the growth and function of neurons. Low levels of BDNF have been linked to depression, and increasing its levels through exercise can help alleviate depressive symptoms. Moreover, the sense of accomplishment and routine that comes with regular exercise can provide structure and purpose, further combating depression.

4. Enhancing Self-Esteem and Body Image

Boosting Self-Confidence

Engaging in regular exercise can significantly enhance self-esteem and self-confidence. Achieving fitness goals, whether it's running a certain distance, lifting a specific weight, or mastering a new yoga pose, fosters a sense of accomplishment. This positive reinforcement builds self-confidence and encourages a positive self-image. The physical changes that come with regular exercise, such as improved muscle tone and weight management, can also contribute to a more favorable perception of oneself.

Positive Body Image

Exercise can improve body image by shifting the focus from aesthetics to functionality and health. Instead of solely aiming for a specific appearance, individuals who exercise regularly often develop an appreciation for what their bodies can achieve. This shift in perspective promotes a healthier, more positive relationship with one's body, reducing the risk of body image issues and related mental health problems.

5. Promoting Better Sleep

Improved Sleep Quality

Exercise has a profound impact on sleep quality, which in turn affects mental health. Physical activity increases the time spent in deep sleep, the most restorative sleep phase. This deeper sleep helps the brain and body recover, leading to improved overall health and well-being. Additionally, regular exercise can help regulate the sleep-wake cycle, making it easier to fall asleep and stay asleep through the night.

Reducing Insomnia and Sleep Disorders

Exercise is particularly beneficial for individuals suffering from insomnia or other sleep disorders. The energy expenditure from physical activity promotes relaxation and reduces the time it takes to fall asleep. Additionally, the mood-enhancing effects of exercise can alleviate anxiety and stress, common contributors to sleep disturbances. By incorporating regular exercise into your routine, you can improve sleep patterns and enhance mental health.

6. Creating a Mindset for Lifelong Wellness

Building Resilience

Regular exercise fosters mental resilience by teaching you to push through physical and mental challenges. The discipline and determination required to maintain an exercise routine translate into other areas of life, helping you cope with stress, setbacks, and adversity. This resilience is a crucial component of mental well-being, enabling you to navigate life's challenges with a positive and proactive mindset.

Establishing Healthy Habits

Engaging in regular exercise helps establish healthy habits that extend beyond physical activity. The routine and discipline of a consistent exercise regimen often lead to other positive lifestyle choices, such as healthy eating, adequate hydration, and prioritizing rest and recovery. These habits collectively contribute to overall wellness, supporting both physical and mental health.

Exercise is a powerful tool for enhancing mental well-being, offering a range of benefits from mood enhancement and stress reduction to improved cognitive function and self-esteem. By understanding and embracing the connection between physical activity and mental health, you can cultivate a mindset and lifestyle that prioritize holistic well-being. Incorporate regular exercise into your daily routine to experience the transformative effects on your mental and emotional health, and enjoy the lifelong benefits of a balanced, active lifestyle.

Techniques for Maintaining a Positive Mindset

Maintaining a positive mindset is crucial for overall well-being and success in various aspects of life. It involves cultivating habits and practices that help you stay optimistic, resilient, and focused, even in the face of challenges. This section delves into effective techniques for developing and sustaining a positive mindset.

1. Practice Gratitude Daily

Keeping a Gratitude Journal

One of the most powerful ways to maintain a positive mindset is by practicing gratitude. Keeping a gratitude journal involves writing down things you are thankful for each day. This practice shifts your focus from what is lacking in your life to the abundance that surrounds you. It can be as simple as acknowledging a sunny day, a kind gesture from a friend, or a personal achievement. By consistently recognizing and appreciating the positive aspects of your life, you train your mind to see the good, which enhances overall happiness and contentment.

Expressing Gratitude to Others

In addition to personal reflection, expressing gratitude to others can significantly boost your positivity. This can be done through verbal appreciation, writing thank-you notes, or performing acts of kindness. Acknowledging the contributions and presence of others not only strengthens your relationships but also reinforces positive interactions and emotions, creating a cycle of goodwill and positivity.

2. Engage in Positive Self-Talk

Reframing Negative Thoughts

Positive self-talk involves consciously transforming negative thoughts into positive ones. When you catch yourself thinking negatively, take a moment to reframe the thought. For example, instead of thinking, "I can't do this," reframe it to, "I will give it my best effort." This shift in perspective can dramatically influence your attitude and approach to challenges. By replacing self-doubt with self-encouragement, you build confidence and resilience.

Affirmations

Affirmations are positive statements that reinforce your goals and values. Repeating affirmations daily can help embed positive beliefs in your subconscious mind. For instance, affirmations like "I am capable of achieving my goals," "I am worthy of love and respect," and "I am resilient and strong" can empower you to maintain a positive outlook. These statements, when repeated regularly, can counteract negative self-talk and foster a more optimistic mindset.

3. Surround Yourself with Positivity

Building a Supportive Network

The people you surround yourself with significantly impact your mindset. Cultivate relationships with individuals who uplift and support you. Engage with friends, family, and colleagues who encourage your growth and well-being. A positive support network provides encouragement during tough times and celebrates your successes, reinforcing a positive mindset.

Limiting Exposure to Negativity

Just as important as surrounding yourself with positive influences is limiting exposure to negativity. This includes reducing time spent with negative individuals, avoiding toxic environments, and being mindful of the media you consume. Negative news and social media can often contribute to stress and pessimism. By curating your environment to minimize negativity, you create a space that fosters positivity and well-being.

4. Practice Mindfulness and Meditation

Mindfulness Exercises

Mindfulness involves being fully present in the moment, without judgment. Practicing mindfulness can help you become more aware of your thoughts and feelings, allowing you to manage them more effectively. Techniques such as deep breathing, body scans, and mindful observation can ground you in the present, reducing anxiety and enhancing your overall sense of calm and positivity.

Meditation

Meditation is a powerful tool for maintaining a positive mindset. Regular meditation practice can reduce stress, increase self-awareness, and promote emotional health. Even a few minutes of meditation each day can help clear your mind and center your thoughts, making it easier to approach life with a positive and balanced perspective. Guided meditations, focusing on themes like gratitude, compassion, and positivity, can be particularly effective in reinforcing a positive mindset.

5. Set Realistic and Achievable Goals

SMART Goals

Setting SMART goals (Specific, Measurable, Achievable, Relevant, Time-bound) helps you maintain a positive mindset by providing clear direction and a sense of purpose. Break down larger goals into smaller, manageable tasks to avoid feeling overwhelmed. Celebrate each milestone you achieve, no matter how small, as this reinforces your progress and keeps you motivated.

Focus on Growth and Learning

Adopt a growth mindset, which emphasizes learning and improvement over perfection. View challenges and setbacks as opportunities for growth rather than failures. This perspective encourages resilience and perseverance, as you understand that each experience contributes to your development. Embracing a growth mindset helps you stay positive and proactive, even when faced with obstacles.

6. Maintain a Healthy Lifestyle

Regular Exercise

Physical activity is closely linked to mental well-being. Regular exercise releases endorphins, reduces stress, and improves mood. Incorporate physical activity into your daily routine, whether it's through structured workouts, recreational sports, or simply taking a walk. The physical benefits of exercise complement the mental benefits, creating a holistic approach to maintaining a positive mindset.

Balanced Diet

Nutrition plays a crucial role in mental health. A balanced diet, rich in vitamins, minerals, and antioxidants, supports brain function and overall well-being. Avoid excessive consumption of processed foods, caffeine, and sugar, as these can negatively impact your mood and energy levels. Prioritize whole foods, hydration, and mindful eating to nourish both your body and mind.

Adequate Sleep

Quality sleep is essential for mental clarity and emotional stability. Establish a consistent sleep routine, create a restful sleep environment, and practice good sleep hygiene. Avoid screens before bedtime, limit caffeine intake, and create a calming pre-sleep ritual. Adequate rest rejuvenates your body and mind, enabling you to approach each day with a refreshed and positive mindset.

7. Engage in Activities You Enjoy

Pursue Hobbies and Interests

Engaging in activities that bring you joy and fulfillment can significantly enhance your positive mindset. Pursue hobbies and interests that allow you to relax, express creativity, and experience pleasure. Whether it's painting, gardening, playing an instrument, or cooking, dedicating time to activities you love fosters a sense of happiness and contentment.

Volunteering and Helping Others

Helping others can be incredibly rewarding and boost your positive outlook. Volunteering your time and skills to support your community or causes you care about creates a sense of purpose and connection. Acts of kindness and service not only benefit those you help but also contribute to your own sense of fulfillment and positivity.

Maintaining a positive mindset requires intentional effort and consistent practice. By incorporating these techniques into your daily life, you can cultivate resilience, optimism, and a proactive approach to challenges. Remember that a positive mindset is not about ignoring difficulties but about approaching them with a constructive and hopeful attitude. Embrace these practices to foster a lasting sense of well-being and create a life filled with positivity and fulfillment.

he Benefits of Mindfulness and Meditation for Fitness

Mindfulness and meditation are powerful tools that can enhance your fitness journey in numerous ways. Integrating these practices into your routine can lead to improved physical performance, mental clarity, and emotional balance. This section delves into the various benefits of mindfulness and meditation for fitness, offering insights into how these practices can transform your approach to exercise and overall well-being.

1. Enhanced Focus and Concentration

Improved Workout Efficiency

Mindfulness and meditation help improve focus and concentration, allowing you to get the most out of your workouts. When you are fully present during exercise, you can concentrate on proper form, breathing techniques, and the specific muscles you are targeting. This heightened awareness ensures that you perform exercises correctly, reducing the risk of injury and maximizing the effectiveness of each movement.

Mind-Muscle Connection

A strong mind-muscle connection is crucial for effective strength training. By practicing mindfulness, you can develop a deeper connection with your body, becoming more attuned to how your muscles feel during each exercise. This connection enhances muscle activation and growth, leading to better results from your workouts.

2. Reduced Stress and Anxiety

Lower Cortisol Levels

Stress and anxiety can negatively impact your fitness progress by increasing cortisol levels, which can lead to weight gain, muscle breakdown, and decreased motivation. Meditation and mindfulness practices have been shown to reduce cortisol levels, helping to manage stress and create a more favorable environment for physical improvement. Lower stress levels also promote better sleep, recovery, and overall health.

Improved Mental Resilience

Mindfulness and meditation cultivate mental resilience, enabling you to handle the challenges and setbacks that often accompany a fitness journey. By developing a calm and centered mindset, you can navigate obstacles with greater ease and maintain a positive attitude. This resilience is particularly beneficial during intense training periods or when facing plateaus in your progress.

3. Better Emotional Regulation

Increased Emotional Awareness

Mindfulness practices enhance emotional awareness, helping you recognize and understand your feelings. This awareness allows you to manage emotions like frustration, disappointment, and self-doubt, which can arise during a fitness journey. By acknowledging and processing these emotions, you can prevent them from derailing your progress and stay committed to your goals.

Enhanced Motivation and Self-Discipline

A mindful approach to fitness fosters greater motivation and self-discipline. Meditation helps you connect with your intrinsic motivations and values, providing a deeper sense of purpose for your workouts. This internal drive makes it easier to stay consistent with your fitness routine, even when external motivation wanes.

4. Improved Recovery and Relaxation

Faster Muscle Recovery

Recovery is a crucial component of any fitness regimen, and mindfulness and meditation can accelerate this process. By promoting relaxation and reducing stress, these practices help lower muscle tension and inflammation, facilitating faster recovery. Incorporating mindfulness into your post-workout routine can enhance the repair and growth of muscle tissues, leading to better performance in subsequent workouts.

Enhanced Sleep Quality

Quality sleep is essential for physical recovery and overall health. Mindfulness and meditation can improve sleep quality by calming the mind and promoting relaxation. Techniques such as deep breathing and progressive muscle relaxation can help you fall asleep faster and enjoy deeper, more restorative sleep. Adequate rest ensures that your body and mind are fully recharged for your next workout.

5. Greater Body Awareness

Listening to Your Body

Mindfulness encourages you to listen to your body and understand its signals. This awareness helps you recognize when you need to rest, when to push harder, and when to adjust your routine to avoid injury. By tuning into your body's needs, you can create a balanced and sustainable fitness regimen that promotes long-term health and well-being.

Injury Prevention

With increased body awareness, you are more likely to notice the early signs of potential injuries. Mindfulness helps you identify areas of discomfort or imbalance before they escalate into more serious issues. By addressing these signs promptly, you can prevent injuries and maintain consistent progress in your fitness journey.

6. Enhanced Performance and Enjoyment

Flow State in Workouts

Mindfulness can help you achieve a flow state during your workouts, where you are fully immersed and engaged in the activity. This state of optimal experience leads to enhanced performance, as you are more focused, motivated, and energized. Achieving flow during exercise also makes the experience more enjoyable, increasing the likelihood that you will stick with your fitness routine.

Greater Enjoyment and Satisfaction

Mindful exercise allows you to appreciate and enjoy the physical sensations and movements of your body. This enjoyment enhances the overall experience, making fitness a pleasurable and rewarding part of your life. By focusing on the present moment, you can derive greater satisfaction from your workouts, reinforcing positive habits and a lifelong commitment to fitness.

7. Mind-Body Integration

Holistic Approach to Fitness

Mindfulness and meditation promote a holistic approach to fitness that integrates the mind and body. This approach recognizes that physical health is deeply connected to mental and emotional well-being. By addressing all aspects of your health, you can achieve a more balanced and fulfilling fitness journey.

Balanced and Sustainable Progress

Mindfulness encourages a balanced perspective on fitness, emphasizing progress over perfection. This mindset helps you set realistic goals, celebrate small victories, and maintain a sustainable pace. By focusing on steady, incremental improvements, you can build lasting habits that support long-term health and wellness.

8. Practical Techniques for Incorporating Mindfulness and Meditation

Mindful Breathing Exercises

Incorporate mindful breathing exercises into your warm-up and cool-down routines. Focus on deep, diaphragmatic breaths to calm your mind and prepare your body for exercise. Mindful breathing can also be used during workouts to maintain focus and regulate your energy levels.

Body Scan Meditation

Practice body scan meditation to develop greater body awareness. This technique involves mentally scanning your body from head to toe, noticing any areas of tension or discomfort. Regular body scans can help you identify and address imbalances, improving your overall physical alignment and performance.

Mindful Movement Practices

Integrate mindful movement practices, such as yoga or tai chi, into your fitness routine. These practices combine physical exercise with mindfulness, enhancing both your physical and mental well-being. Mindful movement can serve as a restorative complement to more intense workouts, promoting flexibility, balance, and relaxation.

By incorporating mindfulness and meditation into your fitness routine, you can experience a wide range of benefits that enhance your physical, mental, and emotional health. These practices foster a deeper connection with your body, improve your performance, and support sustainable progress. Embrace mindfulness and meditation as essential components of your fitness journey to achieve a more balanced, fulfilling, and holistic approach to health and wellness.

Conclusion

Recap of Key Principles and Strategies

As we reach the conclusion of "Fitness Fundamentals: A Beginner's Guide to Effective Exercise," it's essential to reflect on the key principles and strategies we've discussed throughout the book. These foundational elements serve as the building blocks of a successful and sustainable fitness journey.

1. **Setting SMART Goals:**
   - Establishing clear, achievable goals is the first step towards a successful fitness routine. By setting Specific, Measurable, Achievable, Relevant, and Time-bound (SMART) goals, you create a roadmap that guides your efforts and tracks your progress.
2. **Understanding Exercise Principles:**
   - The principles of overload, progression, and specificity are crucial for designing effective workouts. Consistency and recovery are equally important, ensuring that your body adapts and grows stronger over time.
3. **Building a Balanced Routine:**
   - A well-rounded fitness program includes cardiovascular exercise, strength training, flexibility, and balance. Each component plays a vital role in overall health, and together, they create a comprehensive approach to fitness.

4. **Mastering Exercise Techniques:**
   - Proper form and technique are essential to prevent injury and maximize the benefits of each exercise. Warm-up and cool-down routines, along with mindful attention to posture and alignment, enhance your workout's effectiveness.
5. **Incorporating Mindfulness and Meditation:**
   - Mindfulness and meditation improve focus, reduce stress, and foster a deeper connection with your body. These practices support mental and emotional well-being, complementing the physical benefits of exercise.
6. **Maintaining Motivation:**
   - Building a support system, overcoming obstacles, and celebrating progress are key strategies for staying motivated. A positive mindset and accountability are critical in sustaining long-term commitment to fitness.
7. **Integrating Fitness into Daily Life:**
   - Nutrition, hydration, and active living are integral parts of a holistic fitness approach. Incorporating physical activity into your daily routine and finding enjoyable active hobbies ensures that fitness becomes a natural and enjoyable part of your lifestyle.

Encouragement to Continue Your Fitness Journey

Embarking on a fitness journey is a significant and commendable step towards improving your overall health and well-being. The strategies and principles discussed in this book provide a solid foundation, but the true transformation occurs through consistent effort and dedication. Remember that fitness is a lifelong journey, not a destination. Each step you take, no matter how small, brings you closer to your goals and enhances your quality of life.

Celebrate Your Progress:

- Recognize and celebrate the milestones you achieve along the way. Each improvement, whether it's increased strength, better endurance, or improved flexibility, is a testament to your hard work and commitment.

Stay Adaptable:

- Life is dynamic, and your fitness routine should be adaptable to changing circumstances. Be flexible and willing to adjust your goals and strategies as needed, ensuring that fitness remains a positive and sustainable part of your life.

Seek Continuous Improvement:

- Strive for continuous improvement by challenging yourself with new goals and exploring different types of exercise. Variety not only keeps your routine interesting but also ensures comprehensive development and prevents plateaus.

Final Thoughts on the Lifelong Benefits of Staying Active

The benefits of regular physical activity extend far beyond physical fitness. Exercise profoundly impacts mental health, emotional well-being, and overall quality of life. By making fitness a priority, you invest in a healthier, happier future.

Physical Benefits:

- Regular exercise improves cardiovascular health, builds strength, enhances flexibility, and boosts energy levels. It helps manage weight, reduces the risk of chronic diseases, and promotes longevity.

Mental and Emotional Well-Being:

- Exercise is a powerful tool for managing stress, anxiety, and depression. It enhances mood, improves sleep quality, and fosters a sense of accomplishment and confidence.

Enhanced Quality of Life:

- Staying active enables you to enjoy life to the fullest. It enhances your ability to engage in daily activities, pursue hobbies, and maintain independence as you age.